Natural Pregnancy ™

Holistic & Ancient Chinese System For
Getting Pregnant and Having Healthy Babies

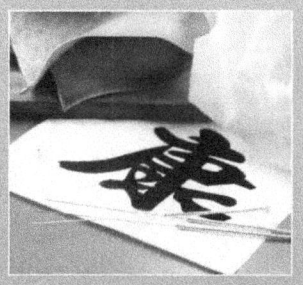

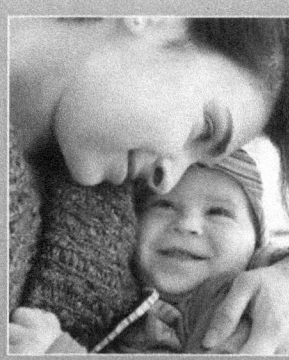

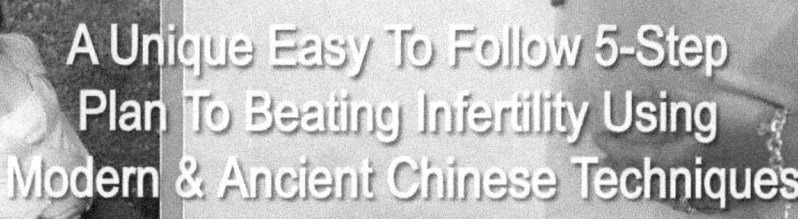

A Unique Easy To Follow 5-Step
Plan To Beating Infertility Using
Modern & Ancient Chinese Techniques

Natural Pregnancy™

A Unique Easy To Follow 5-Step Plan for Beating Infertility Using Modern & Ancient Chinese Techniques

By Dr. Erin Lovett

Copyright Notice

Disclaimer

While all attempts have been made to verify information provided in this publication, neither the Author nor the Publisher assumes any responsibility for errors, omissions or contrary interpretations of the subject matter herein. Any perceived slights of specific persons, peoples or organizations are unintentional. The Author neither makes nor attempts to make any diagnosis or cure or prevent any disease.

This publication is an informational product based on my own experience and research, has not been evaluated by either the FDA or the medical profession and is not aimed to replace any advice you may receive from your medical practitioner. The Author and Publisher assume no responsibility or liability whatsoever on the behalf of any purchaser or reader of these materials. The author is not a doctor, nor does she claim to be. Please consult your primary care physician before beginning any program of nutrition, exercise, or remedy. By consulting your primary care physician, you will have a better opportunity to understand and address your particular symptoms and situation in the most effective ways possible.

As always, before applying any treatment or attempting anything mentioned in this book, or if you are in doubt, you should consult your physician and use your best judgment. If you fail to do so, you are acting at your own risk. You, the buyer or reader of this book, alone assume all risk for anything you may learn from this book. Natural Pregnancy INC, the publisher and Dr. Erin Lovett are not liable or responsible for any increase in severity of your condition or for any health problem you may encounter should you give up medical treatment.

Table of Content

Introduction

From Infertility to Pregnancy

Traveling the Road from Infertility to Motherhood

My story isn't all that unusual. The fact that you're even reading this book tells me one thing: you've suffered like I've suffered. You know what it's like to wish and hope for a baby, trying desperately to conceive only to discover month after month that all of your efforts have been in vain. Your womb is empty and you don't know why. Your arms ache to hold a baby and your heart cries out for a child to call your own.

If you've reached the end of your rope, and wonder if "mommy" is a word that will ever be yelled through the rooms of your home (or only whispered by those who fear to say it too loudly lest they risk upsetting you further), believe me when I say that you can – and will – get pregnant! How do I know this? Because I've been where you are and survived, I've managed to give birth to two healthy, beautiful and smart children after beating the infertility odds.

In some ways my story is unique, and in others it is one of thousands. What makes my story different is its outcome. After years of doing what the medical community suggested, I think – no, I KNOW – that I've found the secrets to helping other women (just like you and just like me), experience the miracle of conception and joy of giving birth. But first, let me tell you a little about my own journey toward motherhood …

Our Story

Like many young newlyweds, my husband and I didn't want children at first. As a matter of fact, we did everything we could to prevent it. But, after five years of marriage, we knew the time had come – we were ready.

With a bit of arrogance (after all, we never thought we couldn't conceive), we jumped headlong into the quest to get pregnant. Only it didn't happen. Why? We wondered after several months. Sure, by now I was in my mid-30's, but I was healthy and strong and had never had any indication that getting pregnant would be a problem once I decided that I was ready for a family.

What should have been easy suddenly became very, very difficult. Being the goal oriented couple we are, my husband and I found it especially difficult to find ourselves on the losing end of our quest. We had never failed at anything before, and let me tell you that this was not something we were prepared to fail at! So we kept trying … and trying … and trying….

Sex was now just that – sex with a purpose. Done when my temperature dictated, it had become a means to an end result, lacking the excitement and the passion it had once held for us.

After more than a year of frustration our relationship began to feel the strain. I was moody and short-tempered, often on the verge of tears. I couldn't bear to watch other women's pregnant bellies grow while mine remained an empty tomb. My every thought revolved around what I was doing (or had done) wrong. What was wrong with me? Why couldn't I do what every other woman could accomplish so easily?

Tired of blaming each other for our inability to conceive we sat down and had a heart to heart talk and decided that it was time to get some answers. After putting off going to the OBGYN for fear of what we'd learn, we decided to face our fears and get tested for a variety of infertility issues.

Unfortunately, like so many other couples discover, the answers we desperately wanted – and needed – weren't going to be available to us. More frustrated than ever, we learned that there was no clear-cut reason for our inability to conceive. Neither of us exhibited any physical, physiological or biochemical reason to prevent a pregnancy. The experts didn't have a clue as to why we weren't pregnant and dubbed us with the term "non-specific infertility." They suggested that we de-stress and keep trying. Great! Hadn't that been what we were doing all along?

That's when I decided to take matters into my own hands. If the experts weren't going to find out what was thwarting our attempts at having a child, I was going to figure it out on my own – and fix it! So, I started to research every aspect of infertility. I read every book and research study I could get my hands on and began talking with hospitals and researchers worldwide about clinical trials and new treatment strategies being considered for couples like us. I was clearly obsessed with my mission and felt as if I'd go nuts if I didn't find an answer.

I began applying all of my newfound knowledge and before long was taking more than a dozen vitamin supplements and minerals every day – and having my husband do the same. I became convinced that pre-conception care for both the husband and wife were the key to conception. We started exercising, eating organic, avoiding toxins wherever we could and even had our amalgam fillings replaced with ceramic to avoid having mercury in our systems. We even began practicing Biorhythmic Lunar Cycle, which shows a woman her most fertile time by comparing the phase of the moon at her birth with the current moon phases.

After four-plus long years of trying anything and everything to get pregnant it worked! We had finally conceived! I couldn't believe my eyes as I stared at those two stripes gleaming from the pregnancy test strip. We'd done it! We were going to have a baby!

Unfortunately, our happiness was short-lived when our precious baby was miscarried at nine weeks. We were devastated. In an instant all of our hopes and dreams had vanished – again!

In the midst of our despair came one glimmer of hope: we had managed to conceive. Our efforts at pre-conception care efforts had worked. Now we had a new hurdle to overcome: carrying a fetus to full term. A mid-wife friend of mine assured me that we were on the right track. We could have a baby, if we kept trying – and learning.

Not long after that conversation, I discovered a very important piece of research. I believe now that it was the final piece to our puzzle and allowed us to not only get pregnant, but to carry our baby to full term – twice! After learning this new "trick" we conceived our daughter within a few short months. Our second pregnancy took less than a month to achieve. Ten years after beginning our quest, we were the proud parents of two beautiful, healthy children!

So what is the secret that we discovered and how did it make the difference to turn us from a desperate infertile couple into proud parents?

We're going to explain everything we've learned in the following pages so that you too can find your way toward the new world that awaits – the world of parenthood!

What This Book Is About and How It Is Organized

Natural Pregnancy isn't your normal pregnancy guide. Sure, it'll teach you about the female and male anatomy and the reasons why so many couples are finding it difficult to conceive these days, as well as offer some traditional help along the way. But there's more.   This guide is designed to take you on the journey of a lifetime; one that goes beyond learning what every doctor out there already knows, in order to help you find your own path to parenthood.

Every couple's story is different, yet every couple's story is the same: they long for a child they can't seem to conceive. If you're one of those couples, this book will show you how to break free from your own infertility issues by learning all the steps needed to attain a Natural Pregnancy of your own:

About Human Anatomy and the Role it Plays in

Infertility Issues

In Chapter One we'll go over the basics of the male and female anatomy including a review of male reproductive organs and the hormonal system; a woman's menstrual cycle; your individual genes; and how they can all affect a couple's fertility; as well as sex and how it can (and should) work when it comes to conceiving a child.

The basics About Infertility

what it is (and isn't); what causes it; who's to blame (and why); the signs to watch out for; how to determine fertility (basal body temperature; cervical mucus; lunar cycles; synchronization) and more ... much more!

The Eastern View of Fertility and the Myths of

Western Medicine

Modern medicine has made great strides in helping infertile couples finally conceive, but does it always work? No! Why? The answer is much simpler than using complicated medications and invasive procedures. Chapter Three will discuss the Eastern World's View on fertility and discuss some of the misconceptions held by traditional medical doctors in regards to fertility and a couple's conception options. This chapter will delve headlong into a discussion on fertility (does it really exist?) and move right into a comparison of both the Eastern and Western views on infertility treatments. Also included will be an in-depth infertility questionnaire for couple's to take to determine their best course of action.

The Steps to Getting Pregnant and Giving Birth to Healthy Children

If getting pregnant and delivering a healthy baby is what you're after, than Chapter Four will offer you the five most important steps to achieving that goal naturally. This includes an in-depth discussion on:

Achieving Balance, Harmony and Congruency for Conceiving Your Baby through a specialized two-step plan that can help enhance any woman's fertility.
Making the Diet and Exercise Changes Necessary to conceive, including vitamin and mineral enhancement; exercising; stress control; sleep optimization and clearing your home and your body of dangerous toxins.
Cleansing Your Energy for Conception Using Acupuncture and Acupressure techniques specifically designed to enhance fertility, as well as tips for balancing your Cycle Phase and Specific Condition with Chinese Herbs and utilizing basic Qi Gong exercises for strengthening your reproductive system and opening the Qi energy pathways needed to conceive.
Internal cleansing and liver detoxification.
Nurturing Your Organs and Enhancing Your Qi Through Acupressure and Qi Gong Exercises.

Within this chapter you will learn the importance of reading your body's signals and signs; keeping a fertility chart; predicting ovulation; and surviving the two-week wait.

Page 20

Special Conditions and Other Infertility Related Disorders

As we've already discussed, no couple's story is exactly the same, which means treating every couple's infertility issues will be slightly different. In Chapter Six we will discuss some of the special circumstances you may be encountering including:

advanced age
unexplained infertility
secondary infertility
mechanical infertility
PCOS, Endometriosis, Fibroids, Ovarian Cysts
Cancer and Infertility
Tubal Ligation
and more ...

Learning More ...

In addition to learning the secrets my husband and I used to conceive our children, we've also decided to add several appendices to the book to discuss other options for couples including In-Vitro Fertilization; Using Yoga and Massage to Conceive; Homeopathic Help; and Healing Both Body and Mind in your quest to conceive.

While some couples may find it beneficial to read the entire book from cover to cover first, and then go back and review sections, which deal with their specific issues and concerns, some couples may opt to begin by reading the sections that best fit their circumstances. How you decide to use the information in this book is certainly up to you, just remember the importance of establishing a complete fertility plan that encompasses a variety of treatment methods to better your chance of having a healthy and happy baby!

Ready to learn more? Great! Let's get started ... boy, do I ever have a lot to tell you ...

Chapter One

All about You and Your Partner's Anatomy and How It Affects Your Fertility

Page 23

If you're worried that chapter one is going to be one big boring health and science lesson, don't. Sure we're going to learn a lot about how our bodies work – and sometimes don't -- but it won't be a repeat of junior high health class. The stuff we're going to learn about now is all the stuff you absolutely need to know in order to get pregnant – and stay pregnant! Let's get started by taking a closer look at the way we are made:

What Makes Her Special

Women are complex creatures – in more ways than one! But nothing may be as complex as her reproductive organs. Here's a quick look at how a woman is capable of bearing children and why it's so important that each organ be in tip-top working order:

The Vagina

Having little to do with your ability to conceive a child, the vagina is considered more of a passageway for the penis and its sperm to enter the opening of the uterus where it can do the job it is intended to do.

One thing that can affect your ability to get pregnant is the hymen, a perforated piece of tissue found at the entrance of the vagina. While the vast majority of young girls have small openings in the hymen, which is later completely torn during the first sexual experience, a small percentage of girls may have an imperforate (or solid) hymen. This can cause blood from the monthly period to back up behind the tissue and into the fallopian tube, which can cause endometriosis, a major factor in female infertility.

The Cervix

The *cervix* is a tight muscle-like tissue found in the lower part of the uterus. Its main job is to hold the baby in place until delivery. However, it also guards against infection by forming a mucus barrier between your vagina and the inside of the uterus.

An incomplete cervix can be a cause for concern, since it is not closed enough to hold the baby in place, thus causing a miscarriage once the baby's weight presses against it, opening the cervix even more. An incompetent cervix can usually be fixed by suturing the cervix closed until delivery.

The Uterus

A woman's uterus, otherwise known as the womb, is typically a pear shaped organ designed to hold and nurture a baby for the nine months it takes to develop inside the mother's body.

In the past it has been highly believed that a woman with a retroverted uterus, or one that is flopped forward toward your pubic bone could not get pregnant. This is simply not true. However, there are some uterine malformations that can affect your ability to both get pregnant and to maintain a pregnancy long enough to give birth to a healthy baby. They include:

A *septate uterus*, which features a band of tissue called the septum which can partially or completely divide the inside of the uterus.

Bicornuate (two-horn) and *unicornuate* (one-horn) uteri feature either one (uni) or two (bi) narrower-than-normal cavities. Women with this type of uterus often miscarry once they do become pregnant.

Polyps, also known as benign fibroid growths in the uterus can interfere with a woman's ability to conceive, and need to be removed in order to increase their chances of an embryo attaching to the uterine wall. Although, removing fibroids can leave scar tissue in the uterine cavity that can make it more difficult to get pregnant since a fetus can have a hard time implanting on scar tissue.

The Ovaries

The ovaries may be two of the most important organs needed to have a baby since they hold and protect the eggs needed for conception. Women do not make eggs throughout their lifetime. Instead, they are born with the amount they will ever have stored in their ovaries. Every month, some are lost due to a variety of biological reasons, while one or two are released for fertilization. If a sperm does not fertilize the egg, it is flushed from the body during the woman's monthly menses. Should one or both ovaries (and the eggs it contains) become damaged or diseased any time during her life, it can greatly affect her chances of ever bearing children.

The Eggs

Without healthy viable eggs, a woman has a zero percent chance of getting pregnant or giving birth to a healthy baby. Eggs are made up of some important factors including its Chromosomes, which contain the genes that will determine what your baby will look and act like; whether it will be short or tall; healthy or not; fat or skinny; and so much more.

A human egg is made up of three protective layers starting with the nourishing and protective cumulus layer; followed by the *corona radiate, a* protective single layer of cells covering the *zona pellucida*, or egg "shell."

A mature, ready-for-fertilization egg (also called an ocycte), contains only 23 chromosomes. Add that to the 23 offered by the male's sperm and your new baby's cells gets the 46 chromosomes needed to be perfect. Miss one or two chromosomes and your baby with either have a serious malady or you will miscarry.

The Fallopian Tubes

Every month a woman's ovaries releases one or two eggs to be fertilized so it can grow in the safety of the womb. But, first, it must get there, travelling by way of the fallopian tube, which connects each ovary to the uterus.

Without healthy tubes, the egg can neither become fertilized (since a blocked tube will prevent the sperm from getting to it in the first place), or make its way to the safety of the nourishing womb. Tubes can be damaged in several ways, with the most common culprits being infection or endometriosis. While both tubes do not have to be clear in order to get pregnant, your chances of conceiving are reduced if one is damaged or blocked in any way.

Her Menstrual Cycle

If all of your reproductive organs are not working properly, they can affect your menstrual cycle and your ability to get pregnant. Unfortunately, when it comes to a woman's menses a lot of things can go wrong. But, before we begin to discuss all of the things that can negatively affect your menstrual cycle, let's first take a look at how it all works:

Step One

A woman's pituitary gland releases FSH -- a follicle-*stimulating hormone* -- after the monthly menses has ended. Meanwhile in the ovary, a dozen or so antral follicles (fluid filled sacs surrounding the egg), begin to grow. It is during this time that at least one egg matures.

In response to FSH and *luteinizing hormone (LH),* the follicle is released by the pituitary gland, and begins to produce *estrogen* in the ovary. At the same time, the estrogen being produced in the ovary signals the uterus to thicken its lining in preparation for the egg's release. This is called the *proliferative phase* of the uterus.

In normal cases, one follicle grows faster than the others, producing more estrogen, causing FSH to decrease and the smaller follicles to stop growing. This signals the pituitary gland to release an *LH surge,* which makes the egg inside the dominant follicle mature.

Step Two

This causes the follicle to burst, releasing the egg which is picked up by one of the fallopian tubes. This is called ovulation.

Step Three

If all goes as planned, the mature egg will meet up with an eager sperm, resulting in an embryo that will now begin to travel down the fallopian tubes, toward the safety of the womb, where it will implant and grow for the next nine months.

Step Four

The leftover part of the follicle, now called the corpus luteum, now begins to produce progesterone, an important chemical to help the embryo implant properly in the lining of the uterus where it can grow. If an egg fails to implant here, the uterine lining will begin to break down and your monthly flow will begin again.

It usually takes about 10-14 days for your body to mature an egg and release it. Ovulation for most women usually takes place between the 10th and 14th day after the start of their last period.

Understanding the importance of consistent ovulation is an important factor in determining why you may be having trouble getting pregnant. For instance, if you are getting your period 12 days or less after you ovulate, you may not be making enough progesterone to support a pregnancy. In contrast, if your cycles are very long, or even irregular, you may not be producing eggs often – or even at all!

Timing Is Everything

Remember, when it comes to getting pregnant, timing is everything, which is why it is so important to understand your menstrual cycle. The biggest mistake a women make is assuming that she is "normal," and so is her ovulation. Most of us have been taught that ovulation occurs around the 14th day so we should be having lots of sex between days 12 and 15. While this may be true for *most* women, it isn't true for *all* women. If you've been trying for awhile to get pregnant, the best thing you may want to look at is exactly when you ovulate and when you're having intercourse.

Ovulation usually occurs 14 days before your period begins. So, if you have a 28 day cycle, then you can expect to ovulate on day 14 like the average woman.

But, if your periods are only 25 days apart, you're going to ovulate around day 11, so having sex on days 13 and 14 will be too late. Conversely, if you have longer periods (say 34 days), you won't even ovulate until day 20, so all that sperm from day 14 and 15 will be long gone by the time it's needed.

To better your chances of getting pregnant, be sure to study your periods; figure out when you actually do ovulate and then make sure that you get busy during the *right* time of the month! For some people, it's that easy!

Of course, it's not always that easy to get pregnant, especially if you have irregular periods. Menstrual cycles that are way off the scale of normal usually indicate an underlining fertility issue such as a lack of regular ovulation, which we'll discuss later. Right now, the important thing is to get in touch with your body and your menstrual cycle so you have the information and knowledge that you'll need as you continue through this book.

What Makes Him the Man You Need To Make a Baby

Like a woman, a man has several important organs needed to create a new life – your baby. Without healthy male reproductive organs even a woman who can easily conceive will not. Now, let's look at some of the things that can affect a man's ability to impregnate his wife:

The Penis

Does size really matter when it comes to getting your gal pregnant? No, not really, as long as the penis is big enough to get the sperm into the vagina and up toward the cervix.

However, function is very important in regards to a male's fertility. Impotence or an inability to either have or sustain an erection can make it difficult to create a pregnancy.

Other problems can occur when the penis is not formed correctly. It is important that the opening that lets the sperm out of the penis be at the
center of the penis' tip. There are two main variations that can cause problems getting pregnant:

Hypospadias – affects about one in 300 men. It is caused when the opening is on the underside of the penis.
Epispadias is caused by the opening at the top of the penis, and is much rarer (only affecting one in 100,000 men).

Both of these conditions are associated with an unusual curvature of the erect penis -- it curves up in epispadias and down in hypospadias — and can prevent the sperm from getting where it's needed in order to fertilize the woman's egg.

The Testicles

A man's testicles both produce and store sperm. It is vitally important for the testicles to be kept a few degrees cooler than 98 degrees for sperm to develop properly. That's why it is so important for men with one testicle larger than the other to be checked for both *hydrocele,* a collection of fluid inside the scrotum; and *varicose,* varicose veins in the testicle, which can both raise testicle temperature and cause infertility.

Unlike a woman's eggs, which are present at birth, a man continues to produce sperm throughout adulthood.

Although produced every day, it does take about two months for a man's sperm to fully mature. The process begins in the testes, where FSH and LH hormones begin making sperm and testosterone. Once the sperm mature in the epididymis, they travel through the vas deferens up to the seminal vesicle and the prostate, where they are submerged in semen and finally ejaculated through the urethra and into the woman's vagina during intercourse.

The Sperm

Without sperm there would be no babies. Without enough of them your chances of becoming pregnant lessen. Every time a man ejaculates, about - 200 million sperm are released. That should certainly be enough to fertilize one little egg now shouldn't it? Maybe not! Within a few hours that 200 million has dwindled to a paltry 100 million. Their job has just gotten harder.

The journey to the egg is long and difficult. First, the sperm needs to know in which direction to swim (statistics show that almost half go in the wrong direction – maybe they should stop and ask for directions!).

Next, they actually have to get moving. Many lag behind. Meanwhile, the woman's body isn't necessarily friendly, killing off thousands of others along the way. For the lucky few, success can be found, but only if they are strong enough and persistent enough to make it through the long arduous journey.

How to Get Together The Right Way: Learning When & How to Do It

As we've already discussed, timing is everything when it comes to getting pregnant. Choose the wrong day to have sex and you'll thwart any efforts at having a baby.

Recognizing the signs of ovulation

There are several ways to tell when you are ovulating:

By watching the calendar (remember, you ovulate 14 days before you get your period)

By watching for an increase in vaginal fluids. Mucus discharge usually becomes heavier, thinner, clearer and stretchy right before and during ovulation.

By feeling inside of your vagina to see when your cervix becomes softer and slightly open. When you are not ovulating, the cervix remains further back in the uterus and feels harder, plus it is tightly closed.

Take notice of any sharp pains in your abdomen or slight spotting around the time you think you will ovulate. While many women do not experience these symptoms, many who do can actually tell when they ovulate. Other physical signs that can indicate ovulation include: headaches; bloating; breast tenderness and pain.

Making Sex Work to Your Advantage

Once you have figured out the best time to have sex to ensure a pregnancy, there are some other simple things you can do to help get the job done:

Lie still for awhile; allowing gravity to help those swimming sperm get to their destination. Avoid going to the bathroom for at least 30 minutes after intercourse.

Place a pillow under your hips after having sex

While many people swear that certain sexual positions can aid the pregnancy quest, others argue that no firm evidence exists to support this notion, so do whatever is comfortable.

Figure out how often to have sex. Too little and you lessen your chances of success; too much and you can deplete your partners' sperm count on the days you need it most. Also keep in mind that waiting as many as five days between love making sessions may help to increase your husband's sperm count, but it can decrease their mobility. But having sex every day will decrease the number of sperm available. So, how often should you be having sex when you're trying to have a baby? Every other day during ovulation seems to be the recommended amount. Most doctors agree that the two days before and the day of ovulation is best, so you may want to do it once on each of those days (but no more than once).

The Role Your Genes Play in Getting Pregnant

Every new baby should get 23 chromosomes from each parent, for a total of 46 chromosomes, arranged in 23 pairs. Less than that (or more than that), and there will be problems. What are your genes? In their most basic form, genes are sections of DNA that occupy certain locations on chromosomes that basically make you "you."

There are four basic types of gene patterns, which, when disrupted can cause serious problems with a pregnancy or a fetus:

Autosomal recessive

If a child inherits an Autosomal recessive gene mutation from both parents, they will get the disease it affects. If both parents carry an Autosomal gene for a specific disease, a child has a 25 percent chance of having the disease, a 50 percent chance of being a carrier of the disease but not having it, and a 25 percent chance of not inheriting the gene at all. Note: Nearly 80 percent of children born with an Autosomal recessive disorder are the first in their family line to have the disease. Why? Because past family members were only gene carriers. Until two carriers of the disease have a child together, the disease can go generations (or even forever) without the disease materializing in offspring.

Autosomal dominant gene

Only one gene transfer from one parent is required for a child to inherit an Autosomal dominant disease.

X-linked dominant gene

An X-linked disease is a mutation of the X chromosome. Girls are more commonly affected simply due to the fact that they carry two X chromosomes. Since men only pass on one X chromosome to their daughters (and never their sons), it is less likely for a boy to inherit an X chromosome dominant disorder.

X-linked recessive gene

As is the case with all recessive genes, both parents must pass it on in order for the child to be affected; either by contracting the disease or being a carrier of the gene mutation.

Genes That Can Limit Your Ability to Get Pregnant

Your genes don't just determine whether you have blue eyes or blond hair; they can also determine whether or not you can get pregnant easily (or at all). Genetic diseases such as Turner Syndrome in women, Klinefelter Syndrome or depletion in the Y chromosome in men can all cause infertility.

As many as 1 in 500 people may also carry a chromosomal translocation, which is a major cause of repeat miscarriage when passed on by either parent.

Thanks to a better understanding of how genes work in relation to getting pregnant and giving birth to a healthy baby, couples can now undergo a series of tests to help them determine if their genes are playing a role in their infertility. While chromosomal testing can be done using several different techniques, the only thing really needed by the parents is a blood sample to determine if either of their chromosomes could be causing a problem.

Page 38

Chapter Two

Understanding Infertility Better

If you and your spouse have been trying to get pregnant for at least a year to no avail, the odds are that you have heard the word infertility at least once from your doctor, friends and family. A scary word to say the least for couples anxious to conceive, but what really is infertility and how do you know if it's something you need to worry about right now?

What is Infertility?

Infertility is basically the inability to get pregnant or to sustain a pregnancy to full term. There are dozens of solid medical reasons why a couple may find conceiving a child or carrying a fetus to full term difficult; leaving them with the dreaded diagnosis of infertility. For some this can be devastating news since without a true reason for their infertility, they feel like there is no way to treat it. While a true diagnosis may make treatment easier for some, not knowing can also be good news since it basically means that there is nothing really "wrong" with either partner.

The goal of this book is to help those suffering from all types of infertility to find new ways to treat their problem in order to finally conceive and give birth to the child they dream of.

What's Causing Your Infertility?

There are literally hundreds of reasons why a couple may be finding it difficult to have a baby. Some are quite simple, like trying at the wrong time of the month; while others may be caused by serious physical ailments and conditions. Most people fall somewhere in between.

The good news is that only about 15% of all couples suffer from any type of infertility; with 1/3 being caused by the man; 1/3 by the woman; and the last third having no known cause. These statistics leave the majority of couples more than able to conceive given enough time and practice. For those who aren't able to conceive within the first year of trying, they'll need to investigate why they are finding having a baby difficult.

It can often take months of testing to discover what the underlying cause of your infertility may be. Women usually begin the process by checking to see if she is ovulating regularly, while men must undergo an initial round of semen testing to ensure that he has sufficient and healthy sperm capable of impregnating his wife.

SIDEBAR: Common Tests for Infertility

To find infertility causes in women, most doctors recommend one or more of the following tests:

Hysterosalpingography

With this test, a dye is injected into the uterus through the vagina, where it will be monitored by x-ray to determine if there are any blockages within the uterus or fallopian tubes which could be hindering a woman's chance of becoming pregnant.

Laparoscopy

An invasive surgical procedure, laparoscopy is used to check the ovaries, fallopian tubes, and uterus for disease and physical problems.

Once your testing is complete, your doctor may discover one or more of the following causes for your infertility issues:

Poor Nutrition: Obesity or anorexia can both cause infertility problems in women.

Endocrine abnormalities: Pituitary, thyroid, or adrenal disorders can all cause infertility.

Vaginal disorders: Abnormalities of the vagina such as stenosis of the vagina or an imperforate hymen may prevent vaginal penetration.

Vaginitis: if severe, may destroy sperm cells.

Cervical abnormalities: Cervisitis polyps may obstruct the canal or, because of associated infection and discharge, may block the transit of spermatozoa through the cervix.

Uterine abnormalities: Any abnormality of the uterus may prohibit egg implantation.

Tubal Obstruction: Tubal obstruction may block the tube, not allowing the egg to make its way to the womb, or the sperm to fertilize it.

Ovarian abnormalities: Congenital abnormalities disturb, disrupt, or destroy ovarian function.

Emotional problems: Severe psychoneurosis or psychosis may inhibit ovulation.

Coital factors: Lubricants, feminine hygiene preparations, or douches, often increase vaginal acidity, which can destroy or inactivate sperm.

Immunologic reaction to sperm

Polycystic ovary syndrome. Nearly 10% of women of child bearing age do not ovulate.

Age. Age may be one of the most frequent causes of infertility as women wait longer and longer to start their families.

Male factors. Low sperm counts, abnormal sperm shape, and low sperm motility are usually asymptomatic conditions to most males.

While most people will find they suffer from one of the infertility factors listed above, some may discover that they suffer from one of the following more serious conditions:

Cervical Hostility to Sperm

For some women, their bodies are not kind to sperm and can actually destroy it. This is called Cervical Hostility. When this is an issue, the man's sperm can not penetrate the cervix properly in order to get to the egg in the uterus.

There are several things that can cause a woman's body to become hostile to her partner's sperm including:

An infection in the lower reproductive tract.
An overabundance of anti-sperm antibodies which can actually immobilize the sperm, preventing it from entering the cervix.

To test for cervical hostility a couple must:

Have intercourse on the two days before ovulation, or on the day of ovulation.
Require the woman to lie on her back for 20 minutes after ejaculation
Have her doctor remove a sample of cervical mucus 8-12 hours after intercourse for closer examination. This will help show the physicians the degree of penetration of the sperm.

If more than 20 actively moving sperm are found per field, cervical hostility is not a concern. If there is less, than further testing is required to determine the cause of the woman's natural hostility toward her husband's sperm.

So, how can you treat for cervical hostility? There are several options:

Antibiotics: This can help clear up any signs of infection.

Estrogen tablets: This can help water down cervical mucus.

IUI and IVF

Steroids: Can be used to stop anti-sperm antibodies from developing. However, they may cause serious side effects.

The Male Factor

Not all infertility issues are due to a woman's inability to conceive or even maintain a pregnancy. Nearly one-third of all cases of infertility experienced by couples are a direct cause of the male's reproductive abilities.

The two most common forms of male infertility are a direct result of a man's lack of sperm. Azospermia, or a complete absence of sperm can completely inhibit a couple's chance of conceiving a baby, while oligospermia (a low sperm count of less than 20 million sperm per ml), can make it very difficult – if not impossible – to have a baby without medical intervention.

For some couples suffering with these conditions, donor sperm is needed to conceive a child, although some men can be treated with oral testosterone to increase their sperm supplies.

Retrograde ejaculation is another concern that can affect a man's ability to father a child, since semen enters the bladder instead of emerging through the penis during orgasm, thus preventing sperm from getting where it needs to be to fertilize his partner's egg.

Hypospadia is a birth defect which causes the urethra to exit the penis closer to the base, rather than at the tip of the penis, causing impotence.

Infertility in Women

Of course, women can suffer from a variety of infertility issues too including:

Anovulation

An absence of ovulation which can be caused by:

Stress

Chronic mental illness, such as depression.

Chronic physical illness, such as inflammatory bowel disease, poorly controlled diabetes, tuberculosis or anemia.

Under nutrition or inadequate body fat.

Prolonged or continuous physical exertion.

Various pharmaceutical or recreational drug use.

Hormone imbalances.

Pituitary or ovarian failure.

Infertility due to tubal damage

One of the main causes of female infertility, tubal disease, is a disorder in which the fallopian tubes are blocked or damaged in some manner. There are a number of treatment options available to overcome infertility caused by tubal disease including:

Surgical removal of scar tissue
Surgical repair of damaged tubes

Tubal ligation reversal

In-vitro fertilization or IVF

Infertility due to Recurrent Pregnancy Loss

A miscarriage is considered a pregnancy loss under a 20 week gestation. To be deemed a recurrent miscarriage candidate, you must have had at least three miscarriages.

Although recurrent pregnancy loss is considered a form of infertility, miscarriage itself is not. As a matter of fact nearly half of all pregnancies end in early miscarriage (most before the woman ever knows she is pregnant), and 20% or so (nearly one in every 5- 6 pregnancies) end in a miscarriage between the first and fourth months. There are a lot of reasons for a miscarriage. Here are just a few of the most common:

Chromosomal abnormalities in the fetus. It is estimated that 7 out of 10 pregnancies that end in miscarriage before the 12th week are due to some sort of chromosomal abnormality in the fetus.

Genetic factors. Translocation in the parents can be a contributing factor to recurring miscarriage, especially when there is a family tendency toward lost pregnancies.

Environmental factors. Exposure to noxious or toxic substances are known to be associated with recurrent miscarriages as are social drugs, cigarettes, alcohol and larger amounts of ingested caffeine. Even anesthetic gases, dry cleaning fluids, petroleum products and some medications used to treat acne can cause recurring miscarriage in users.

Medical conditions. Uncontrolled Diabetes and Thyroid disease may make it more difficult to maintain a pregnancy in some women.

Auto immune disease. As many as one in ten women with recurrent miscarriages show some evidence of auto immune factors.

Structural defects: Uterine septum or adhesions can all make it difficult to carry a baby to full term.

What Causes Infertility	
Factor	Percentage of cases
Male : Defective sperm production	30-40 %
Female: Ovulation Issues	5-25%
Tubal or uterine Problems	15-25%
Cervical/immunological Issues	5-10%
Unexplained Reasons for infertility	10-25%

Knowing When You Are Most Ready to Make a Baby: Knowing the Signs of Fertility

As we've already discussed, knowing exactly when you ovulate can definitely make a difference between getting pregnant and not getting pregnant. That's why it is so important to watch for those natural signs that can point you toward the right moment to try and make your baby. Here are some of the most basic road signs to watch for on your journey toward parenthood:

Cervical Mucus Changes

Every woman experiences a certain degree of vaginal discharge all of the time, But, taking note of how that discharge, or cervical mucus, changes throughout the month, can be a good indicator as to when you ovulate, and thus, when you should try to conceive a child.

The texture and the consistency of cervical mucus changes throughout the month. The closer ovulation gets, your cervical mucus will change from a creamy look and texture to a clear, very stretchy texture that is wetter than you'll notice at other times of the month. Here are the basic stages your cervical mucus will undergo throughout the month:

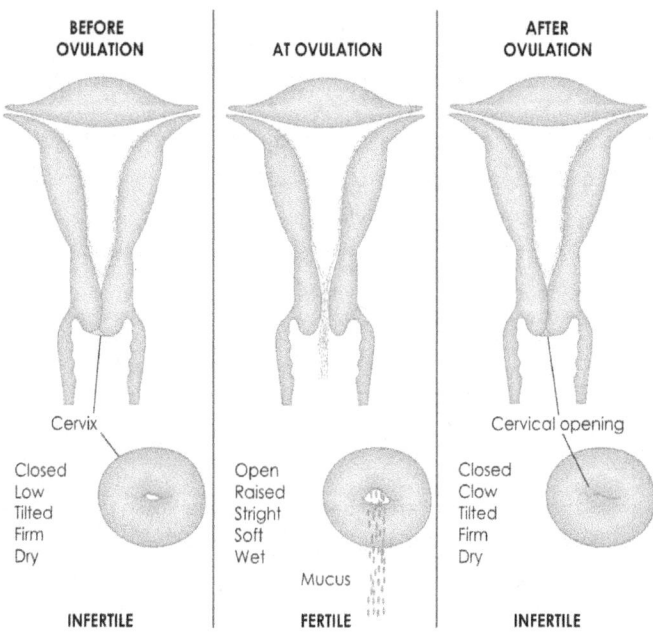

The Infertile phase

Right after your period ends, you may experience several "dry" days with no visible mucus. This is your infertile time of the month.

The Fertile phase

As ovulation nears, you'll begin to feel cervical mucus seeping from the vagina. It will appear moist and sticky at first and may be white or a creamy color. When tested with your finger it will hold its shape and break easily.

As you get closer to ovulation, this mucus will begin to change; increasing in amounts and becoming cloudier and become stretchy when finger tested.

As your body begins to increase its estrogen production, you will experience a much "wetter" sensation around the vulva, with the mucus increasing in volume. At this point it should look like a raw egg -- white, thin, watery and transparent. When tested, it may now stretch for several inches before breaking. This is considered high fertile mucus, allowing sperm to live several days.

Your Peak Day

Peak day is considered the LAST day that you can see or feel this highly fertile-type slippery, transparent, stretchy mucus. While it sometimes coincides with ovulation, it usually follows ovulation within a day or two.

This is the best time to try and get pregnant since this highly fertile mucus ensures that **fresh, healthy sperm** are ready to meet **a fresh, healthy egg as soon as ovulation occurs.**

Post-ovulatory completely infertile phase

Right after your peak day, that slippery sensation will cease and your mucus will become sticky and dry once again. This is due to an increase in progesterone production, which thickens the mucus to form a plug at the cervix and prevent sperm from entering during the wrong time of the month.

Checking Your Cervical Mucus

The easiest way to check your cervical mucus is when you go to the bathroom. But, be sure to use your finger and not toilet paper, which will absorb some of the moisture.

Note: It's also important to check the mouth of the vagina, not the walls (since they are always moist).

If you are finding it difficult to tell the difference between cervical mucus and normal vaginal secretions try this simple test:

Dip a sample of mucus (or secretion) into some water. If it forms a blob and sinks, it is cervical mucus, but if it dissolves, it is a normal secretion.

Tips for Observing Mucus Changes

For most women, checking for changes in their cervical mucus isn't difficult, once they know what they're looking for. Here are some examples of how the mucus may feel during its different stages:

Dry: It feels the same as when you rub your fingers over the lips on your face or rub your arm.
Wet: Similar to the feeling of rubbing your tongue over your lips or even wetting your arm and rubbing it.
Slippery Wet: See how it feels to put lip gloss on your lips, and then rub your tongue over them, or put hand cream or aloe Vera gel on your arm and rub it. Or better yet, touch a fish in water.

When checking your mucus it will look

and feel like this:

Moist or Sticky (early mucus): scanty, thick and white (holds its shape).

Wetter (transitional mucus): more abundant, thinner, cloudy and stretchy.

Slippery (highly fertile mucus): profuse, thin, transparent and very stretchy (resembles a raw egg).

Sensation at the Vulva	Finger Test	Appearance
Moist or Sticky		**Early Mucus** Scanty Thick White Sticky Holds its shape
Wetter		**Transitional Mucus** Increasing Amounts Thinner Cloudy Slighty Stretchy
Slippery		**Highly Fertile Mucus** Profuse Thin Transparent Stretchy (like raw egg white)

Basal Body Temperature

If you've been trying to get pregnant for any length of time, the odds are that you already know about your Basal Body Temperature (BBT). It is considered the best way to determine the best time to have sex to ensure a pregnancy or to determine if you may suffer from a luteal phase defect.

What is your Basal Body Temperature? The temperature of your body at rest. Taking your temperature right away in the morning before you do anything (getting out of bed, eating, drinking or even going to the bathroom), is essential to getting an accurate reading. While you don't need a special thermometer to chart your BBT, investing in a BBT thermometer that registers degrees within 1/10th can be very helpful.

Once you begin to chart your morning temperatures, you will begin to see definite changes throughout your cycle. This will help you figure out when you ovulate. Be sure to take your reading at the same time each day, and remember illness or not getting enough sleep can affect it. Generally speaking most women experience slight fluctuations in their temperature (by about 1/10th of a degree) from day to day.   When your temperature rises .2 degrees higher than any temperature taken in the last 6 days, and it stays elevated for three consecutive days, you can usually assume that you have ovulated.   By tracking this temperature rise for several months, you should be able to predict when you ovulate each month. In the event that you are not ovulating, your temperature will remain stable, giving you a red flag to discuss with your doctor.

Simple Steps to Charting Your BBT

You know the importance of charting your Basal Body temperature, but what's the best and easiest way to ensure that you're doing it correctly? Try following these simple steps:

First, get the right instrument – glass basal body thermometers are BEST.

Begin on the first day of your temperature (use the attached chart).

Be sure to shake down the thermometer before you go to bed.

As soon as you wake up in the morning, take your temperature for 5 minutes before getting out of bed, smoking, eating, or drinking.

Record your temperature on the chart by placing a black dot on the temperature line in the correct date column.

Draw a line between yesterday's temperature dot and today's dot.

Mark days you have sex by circling the dot.

Record any reasons for temperature fluctuations (a cold, fever, medications or even a lack of sleep) with a star.

Start a new chart the day your period begins.

Charting Your Temperature

The easiest way to chart your BBT is to use a series of dots placed on the graph. Start by placing a dot on the graph on the spot corresponding to each day's temperature. Join the dots of consecutive days. If you do not take your temperature one day, do not join the dots across that day. Also write out the temperature numerically in the space provided.

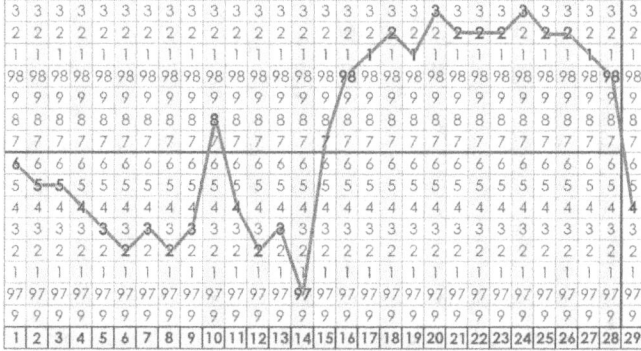

Why does the temperature rise?

As we have already discussed, Ovulation causes your progesterone levels to rise, which generates more body heat. This is what causes the BBT to increase. Your temperature won't (and can't) go up without ovulation, so be sure to look for a strong prolonged rise.

Here are some of the most common scenarios to watch out for when charting your Basal Body temperature:

A Sloping Rise: Temperatures do not have to change abruptly to indicate ovulation. A gradual incline (or sloping rise) is sufficient. Watch for a gentle curve over a three to four day time span as the temperature rises to indicate ovulation.

A Slow Rise: Similar to a sloping rise, a slow rise may be indicated by a steady shift of temperature in small increments of one tenth of a degree Fahrenheit over a 4-5 day period.

A Fallback Rise: In a fallback rise pattern the temperature rises significantly and abruptly as you would expect, followed by a dip before rising again and remaining higher throughout the luteal menstrual phase.

A Staircase Rise: When temperatures rise in a staircase pattern, it stays steady or may even slightly decrease and then rise and stay steady again until reaching the elevated level. This can take a couple of days.

Triphasic Charting: Showing three levels of temperatures (pre-ovulation; ovulation; and post ovulation), A Triphasic chart is usually used to detect pregnancy.

Cervical Palpation

Watching for changes in your cervix's position can also indicate ovulation – or a lack of it. Depending on the time of the month, your cervix may feel firm and dry and easy to reach. It will also feel closed. Closer to ovulation, it will become softer, wetter and get harder to reach as it pulls further up into your uterus. Plus, it will feel open to the touch, allowing the sperm to make their way through. When it is the softest and hardest to reach, you are ovulating.

Cervix & Mucus

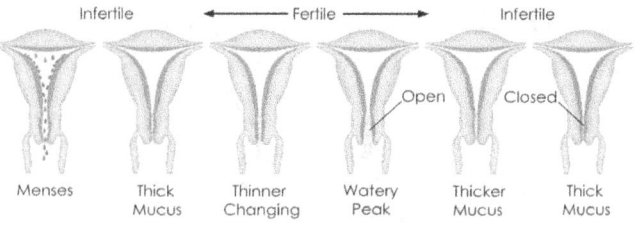

Checking Your Cervix

Checking your cervix isn't difficult, although you do need to know what signs you are looking for and how it should feel.

Don't worry about your hands being sterile, washing them is good enough.

The first thing you'll be looking for is the firmness (or hardness) of the cervix. Since ovulation tends to soften the cervix, this is an excellent indicator of ovulation and can help you determine your most fertile time of the month.

Next, you'll want to check the position of your cervix (how high or low it is). As ovulation approaches it can rise as much as an inch into your pelvis, lowering again after ovulation.

Lastly, you'll want to see how open or closed your cervix is during each phase of your cycle. The opening of the cervix begins to open with ovulation (you'll actually be able to stick your finger through it).

So, how do you check each of these items? Start by using the same position each time (putting one foot on a low stool is best) and inserting your finger all the way into your vagina (reaching up and back) until you feel the top.

Your cervix can be felt on the underside of the tip of your finger. If you do not feel your cervix, try pressing on your lower abdomen. Just be sure to do this each time you do a cervix check since consistency is vital for accurate charting.

Next, place each of your fingers on opposite sides of the cervix and bring them together to gather any mucus that may be on the cervix. Be sure not to squeeze the cervix. While gathering the mucus, observe your cervix's firmness, position, and openness. Draw your closed fingers out and check any mucus you have recovered using the suggestions mentioned earlier.

When You Shouldn't Check The Cervix

Never check your cervix during menstruation. Not only will you be unable to detect fertile signs at this time, you may introduce infection to the area.

Other times you should not check your cervix include:

Right after you get up from your night's sleep or from a long nap. Why? The cervix tends to be consistently higher when first rising.
Right after a bowel movement – it can change its position.
If you have a number two or higher pap smear, discontinue the cervical check until your cervix returns to normal.
If you have an active outbreak of genital herpes or genital warts.

When checking your cervix, **Peak Day** is defined as the *last* day of any fertile sign including: slippery mucus or slippery feeling *or a* low, soft, or open cervix. This is a good time for intercourse.

How to Chart Cervical Changes

Any change may indicate fertility, so be sure to learn what your infertile cervix feels like in order to determine when fertility changes occur. This can take 1-3

Page 63

cycles of observation. That's why it's so important to chart your cervical changes properly.

Be as consistent with your observations and charting as possible to enable you to better see the patterns of your fertile cervix.

It is easiest to *draw* the changes of the cervix on a chart. Use a dot to signify a closed cervix; a circle for an open cervix.

If the cervix is low in the vaginal canal, draw it low in the space for cervical observations. If the cervix is high up the vaginal canal, draw it higher up in the space for cervical observations.

If cervical mucus is present, add the word **mucus** or **slippery** to the box for cervical mucus observations. Next, write **Firm** if the cervix is firm and **Soft** if the cervix is soft.

Lunar Cycle

Lunar fertility is based on the assumption that each woman's menstrual cycle and individual periods of fertility are directly influenced by the phases of the moon. While not for everyone, those who firmly believe in astrology and the affects it can have on our bodies and health may find lunar cycling a positive way to enhance their fertility.

Most healthy women experience a menstrual cycle that is equal to one lunar month, or 29 days. In addition, the average length of a full term pregnancy is exactly 9 lunar months, or 38 weeks.

It is reported that the moon can affect the menstrual cycle by:
regulating it
triggering ovulation
affecting emotions
affecting behavior

How Lunar Cycling Works

The appearance of the moon changes each day depending on how it orbits the earth and where it is positioned in regards to the sun. It takes 28 days to go through one entire cycle. The lunar fertility theory implies that a woman is most fertile during the same lunar phase as the day she was born. Using this premise, a specially trained astrologers can pinpoint the time and date at which an individual woman is most fertile each month.

How to use the lunar cycle for fertility enhancement?

Using the lunar cycle to increase your chances of getting pregnant is pretty simple. Basically it works like this: if you were born 3 days before a full moon, then you will be most fertile 3 days before each full moon.

Calculating your lunar cycle

While it is usually best to have an experienced astrology consultant determine your cycle, it is possible to do it yourself.

The first step is determining your natal age. To do this you will need to know the time, date and place of your birth. Let's assume that you were born when the angle between the sun and the moon was 60 degrees, or about 5 days after the crescent or new moon. This will make your most fertile time about 5 days after each new moon. Of course fertility can be experienced for a brief time before and after this day. All you need to know is your natal angle (for example 60 deg.), when it occurs in the lunar month (for example, 5 days after a new moon) and on which dates this recurs each calendar month.

Synchronization

How does synchronization affect a woman's menstrual cycles? By allowing her to give off pheromones, an airborne chemical that signals your mate that you are ready biologically for sex and reproduction. While it is best to have your hormonal cycle synchronized with your personal lunar rhythm, it doesn't always work like that.

Which cycle shifts?

Your lunar cycle is, of course fixed, which is not the case for your hormonal cycle. It can be affected by a number of outside influences including stress, trauma, travel, health, weight changes and more. This can all affect when you ovulate.

To synchronize your menstrual cycle, you need to reprogram it using both your conscious and subconscious.

To work on your conscious mind you will need to:

Become more aware of the hormonal rhythms of your body
Avoid situations which can change your hormonal cycle (stress, diet, sudden changes in your environment, etc)
Chart your lunar peak dates.

Working on your subconscious may be a bit more difficult since it requires maintaining a relaxed alpha state as often as possible in order to synchronize your hormonal cycle with your natural lunar cycle so you can identify your fertile time more easily.

Female Hormone Factors

Every woman knows that her hormones rule her body. This is especially true when it comes to making a baby. Without just the right amount of specific hormones released at certain times of the month, a woman doesn't stand a chance of either conceiving a baby, let alone carrying one to full term. Here is a quick overview of the hormones needed to achieve and maintain a pregnancy:

Hormone to Test	Time to Test	Normal Values	What Value Means
Follicle Stimulating Hormone (FSH)	Day 3	3-20 mIU/ml	Under 6 is considered excellent, 6-9 is good, 9-10 fair, 10-13 diminished ovarian reserve, 13+ means very hard to stimulate which may cause infertility
Estradiol (E2)	Day 3	25-75 pg/ml	A high level of E2 may indicate the presence of a functional cyst or diminished ovarian reserve.
Estradiol (E2)	Day 4-5 of meds	100+ pg/ml or 2x Day 3	Since the number of follicles a woman has can determine her E2 levels during ovarian stimulation, most doctors look for an increase as an indication that ovulation is occurring. However, some doctors prefer to use a formula of either 100 pg/ml after 4 days of stims, or a doubling in E2 from the level taken on cycle day 3.
Estradiol (E2)	Surge/hCG day	200 + pg/ml	The levels should be 200-600 per mature (18 mm) follicle...

Hormone to Test	Time	Normal	What Value Means

	to Test	Values	
Luteinizing Hormone (LH)	Day 3	< 7 mIU/ml	A high level of LH may indicate PCOS.
Luteinizing Hormone (LH)	Surge Day	> 20 mIU/ml	An LH surge indicates that ovulation will occur in the next 48 hours
Prolactin	Day 3	< 24 ng/ml	Increased prolactin levels can interfere with ovulation...
Progesterone (P4)	Day 3	< 1.5 ng/ml	An elevated Progesterone level may inhibit pregnancy.
Progesterone (P4)	7 dpo	> 15 ng/ml	A progesterone test is done to confirm ovulation. A level over 5 probably indicates some form of ovulation, but a level over 10 is preferred for normal ovulatory function.
Thyroid Stimulating Hormone (TSH)	Day 3	.4-4 uIU/ml	Mid-range normal in most labs is about 1.7. A high level of TSH combined with a low or normal T4 level generally indicates hypothyroidism.
Free Triodothyronine (T3)	Day 3	1.4-4.4 pg/ml	IN the event the thyroid gland is still producing normal levels of T4, a T3 test will help determine an ineffective thyroid. accurate evaluation of thyroid function.
Free Thyroxin (T4)	Day 3	.8-2 ng/dl	A low level of T4 may indicate a diseased thyroid gland or non-

functioning pituitary gland which is not stimulating the thyroid to produce T4.

Hormone to Test	Time	Normal	What Value Means
Total Testosterone	Day 3	6-86 ng/dl	A level above 50 is considered abnormal.
Free Testosterone	Day 3	.7-3.6 pg/ml	

	to Test	Values	
Dehydroepiandrosterone Sulfate (DHEAS)	Day 3	35-430 ug/dl	
Androstenedione	Day 3	.7-3.1 ng/ml	
Sex Hormone Binding Globulin (SHBG)	Day 3	18-114 nmol/l	Increased androgen production often leads to lower SHBG
17 Hydroxyprogesterone	Day 3	20-100 ng/dl	Mid-cycle peak would be 100-250 ng/dl, luteal phase 100-500 ng/dl
Fasting Insulin	8-16 hours fasting	< 30 mIU/ml	. Fasting insulin of 10-13 generally indicates some insulin resistance, and levels above 13 indicate greater insulin resistance.

Blood Glucose Levels			
Type of Test	Time to Test	Normal Values	What value means
Fasting Glucose	8-16 hours fasting	70-110 mg/dl	A healthy fasting glucose level is between 70-90, but up to 110 is within normal limits. A level of 111-125 indicates impaired glucose tolerance/insulin resistance. A fasting level of 126+ indicates type II diabetes.
Glycohemoglobin / Glycosylated Hemoglobin (HbA1c)	anytime	< 6 %	An HbA1c measures glucose levels over the past 3 months should be under 6% to show good diabetic control (postprandial glucose levels rarely going above 120), which reduces the risk of miscarriage and birth defects.

Having Your Spouse's Semen Checked

In order to determine if your partner's semen contains enough healthy sperm to get you pregnant, a semen analysis is required. This involves a trip into the doctor's office where he will be asked to ejaculate into a testing cup.

Note: for the most accurate results it is important that he refrain from any type of ejaculation for 2-5 days prior to the test!

The first thing the doctor will look at is whether or not your spouse's sperm look normal. This includes checking the head, the midpiece and the tail for abnormalities. Some problems that may be discovered during this stage of testing are:

An Abnormal Head:

Since the head of the sperm holds all of its genetic makeup, a round, pinhead, large head or double head can't fertilize an egg.

Page 74

Fructose Deficiency

Fructose is necessary to give the sperm enough energy to move from the cervix to the uterus. If the midpiece does not contain a sufficient supply of fructose, it won't be able to make the long journey ahead.

A Malformed Tail

Sperm with no tail, two tails, or coiled tails do have the propulsion capability needed to get to the egg for fertilization.

The World Health Organization (WHO) has set some standard parameters for determining a sperm's normalcy. In order to be considered A-plus sperm capable of fertilizing a female egg with no problems, a man's sperm must meet the following criteria:

Volume: Should be 1.5 to 5 ml, or approximately a teaspoon.
Concentration: Should be greater than 20 million sperm/ml, or a total of greater than 40 million per ejaculate.
Motility: More than 40 percent of the sperm should be motile, or moving.
Morphology: More than 30 percent of a man's sperm should be normally shaped, according to the WHO criteria, however, some doctors follow more stringent parameters (as listed below) to determine fertility. A score of at least 14% is needed to be considered normal; 4-13% for a borderline diagnosis; with less than 4% being considered poor fertility.

This more stringent criterion requires the following evaluation:

Forward progression of sperm: On a scale of 1 to 4, sperm needs to be grade at least a 2-plus, meaning the sperm moves forward adequately.
White blood cells: Should be no more than 0 to 5 per high-power field.

Hyper viscosity: Should gel promptly but liquefy within 30 minutes after ejaculation.

Ph Levels: Should be alkaline – this protects sperm from vaginal acid.

HOS, or hypo-osmotic swelling, test: To determine normal function, more than 50 percent of the sperm tails should swell when exposed to a hypo-osmotic solution.

Antisperm antibodies: If antisperm antibodies are present, they can attach themselves to the sperm tail, interfering with movement.

Acrosome reaction test: The head of the sperm is covered with two layers of membranes, called the *Acrosome* that contain enzymes which help it penetrate the egg. Without an "acrosome reaction" penetration is impossible, so this reaction is tested to determine fertility.

Making Love = Making Babies

It may seem obvious, but too many couples who are having difficulty getting pregnant forget the #1 rule to conceiving a child: having sex! Believe it or not, more than half of all couples trying to have a baby have sex less than once a week.

True, your libido can take a hit from a lot of things including age, health and the stress of trying to overcome fertility issues, but the fact remains: making love = making babies, and without lots of sex you lessen your chances of conceiving even more!

For many couples, sex is considered something of an exploding passion, during softer, deeper intercourse that lasts thirty minutes or more can make it easier to conceive by allowing the couple to experience true love and peace; an important ingredient to making a baby.

Chapter Three

Taking a New Look at Fertility: How the East and West Differ in Their Views and How It Can Help You Get the Baby You Dream Of

Traditionally, a couple has been considered infertile after a year of trying to conceive with no luck. If the term "infertility" leaves you terrified of never becoming parents, relax: some experts actually argue that infertility doesn't even exist! Are you feeling a little less fearful and little more hopeful after hearing that? Good! That's what this book is all about. Now, let me explain …

Does Infertility Even Exist?

There are a lot of things that can impede a couple's ability to conceive a child, but unless a woman's reproductive organs are damaged in some way, she shouldn't be told that she can't conceive, because she can (with of course, a little help). Although conception can be more difficult for some, it is usually possible, although it could a bit more time and assistance than normal.

Of course, getting the help you need to conceive can be expensive, especially when relying on traditional methods offered by modern science. Thankfully, today's high-tech (and high-priced) medical advances aren't the only ways to enhance a couple's fertility. There are plenty of more natural ways to fix a fertility issue. People all over the world have been using a variety of more homeopathic ways to enhance fertility in both men and women – not to mention fix "plumbing problems."

If you are anxious to conceive, but have been dealing with delays, now's the time to look at ALL of your options. The good news is that the vast majority of you reading right now *can* conceive. It's just going to take some perseverance in finding the right approach, but it can (and will) happen.

The two most common views of fertility come from two opposite arts of the earth: The East and the West. Now, let's take a closer look at these two worldviews differ when it comes to treating infertility:

Understanding How the East Looks At Fertility

The entire basis of the Eastern view of medicine relies on the fact that every health issue (including fertility) is directly tied to his/her environment. Cause and effect are the mainstay beliefs of Eastern medicinal views.

The Chinese believe that the entire human body is a complex eco-system, with even the smallest part affecting all others. They never disregard how some part of the body may be affecting another. This is why they strive so hard for complete balance within all systems; including the body's organs, fluids and even its energy supplies. If just a single thing is out of whack it can cause serious problems – especially when it comes to conceiving a child!

Instead of treating a problem, the Chinese believe in treating the whole body. By balancing every part of the body, the Chinese method of healing is able to coax the body to function more efficiently. For a woman trying to conceive, this requires taking a good hard look at a woman's overall health and well being (including her physical, emotional and spiritual state of mind), looking for anything that could be disrupting her ability to conceive.

Once found, treatment may include changing her diet, exercise plan, adding herbal supplements or undergoing acupuncture (and more) in order to make conception possible.

Page 81

The Basics of Traditional Chinese Medicine

Traditional Chinese Medicine was founded on the philosophy of Tao, or an interplay of opposites. Most people know this as the Yin and the Yang. What is the Yin and the yang and why is it important to your fertility? Yin and Yang are opposite types of energy (one positive and one negative). However, they both contain small bits of the other, making it very important that they each are balanced in the body. Otherwise, chaos can erupt, causing disease and afflictions.

According to Chinese philosophy, everything we do, eat and think affects the balance of these two energies and if perfect health is to be achieved and equal balance of the Yin and the Yang must be maintained. By balancing what we eat, how we act and think and what we do from day to day, we can – and will— determine how healthy our bodies remain. When we work too hard without enough rest, our physical and mental well being begins to suffer. Suddenly we catch a cold or the flu. We feel tired and drained and can't seem to catch up. An excess in one of these energies causes a deficiency in another. Fertility is especially sensitive to shifts in these two energies. How? Let's take a closer look.

The Yin is responsible for getting the uterus ready to take care of a fertilized egg. It creates the estrogen needed to produce a thick uterine lining, cervical changes and mucus necessary for a fertilized egg to be nourished and grow inside a woman's body. As we age, this Yin energy diminishes, causing the Yang (or hot energy) to take over. It's this drop in estrogen levels (your Yin energy) and rise in Yang energy that causes hot flashes and night sweats during menopause. When an aging woman wants to become pregnant, she needs to increase her Yin and decrease her Yang to better her chances of conceiving. Of course, that is only one simple example of how the Yin and Yang affect fertility. Let's investigate further.

QI: The Energy of Life

The energy within our bodies flows like electricity. Every cell conducts and transfers it through protein molecules. This invigorates and powers our internal organs, which in turn directs every chemical and hormonal release within each bodily system. This is what the Chinese call "Qi."

The Qi flows through a network of channels called meridians. It is these meridians that acupuncturists use to redirect lost and misguided energy in the body.

The Yin, Yang and blood are all types of Qi that carry energy throughout the body and take away waste products.

The third form of Qi, your organs and systems, also work together to keep your body in equal harmony. While traditional western medicine may only look at one system at a time to develop a therapy treatment, Eastern medicine requires taking all forms of the Qi into account when trying to heal a specific problem. For instance, a woman with a menstrual issue may find herself being treated for a liver ailment by a Chinese practitioner, thus solving her fertility issue via the liver. This is because the Chinese medical community investigates the interaction between all organs and bodily systems at all times due to the reliance of the Qi.

The Organs

There are six pairs of meridians that relate to specific organ systems:

The Heart

The Lung & Large Intestines (this does not affect fertility)

The Kidneys

The Spleen, Digestion and Immunology Systems

The Liver and Gallbladder

The Uterus

The Heart and Spirit

According to Chinese philosophy, the heart does much more than circulate blood through the body. It also affects the mind and spirit, which creates our personality which helps us to find peace with our circumstances. When looking at the heart in terms of fertility, consider this: Since the heart is responsible for providing the necessary blood flow to the uterus, any type of emotional upset which affects the heart and spirit can disrupt the uterus's ability to nourish and develop a fetus.

The first thing a Chinese practitioner will likely consider when treating a woman for fertility issues is to look at a disturbance in her Uterine Vessel, called the Bao Mai. This is an important link between the heart and the uterus. Women who do not have regular periods often suffer with a Bao Mai blockage that needs to be treated.

The Kidneys

Traditionally considered responsible for the elimination of waste products and the body's water balance, Chinese medicine also attributes a person's genetic makeup to the kidneys. This means that it is the kidneys that dictate when a girl will begin menstruating; when a woman will enter menopause and what happens in the years in between.

According to Traditional Chinese Medicine philosophy, the kidneys connect and encompass other important organs and systems including: the reproductive organs; skeletal system; neurologic system and the endocrine system.

So, how does this help to treat infertility? For some women (especially older ones), stimulating the kidney system can restore normal levels of FSH used to stimulate the ovaries to produce more estrogen, and develop healthier follicles and eggs needed for conception. Of course the use of herbs and acupuncture can also help to revitalize the kidneys and alleviate infertility caused by weak kidneys.

The Spleen, Digestion and Immunological Systems

The spleen's job is simple according to modern medicine: produce and destroy blood and immune cells. Chinese medicine however, gives the spleen a more important job – to oversee the energy within the body. Transforming food into Qi; blood into energy; the spleen is very important when it comes to keeping every organ in the body working in sync. Since it is also responsible for producing several hormones, an inactive or improperly acting spleen can impact a woman's ability to conceive and carry a baby to full term.

Things that can damage a spleen and keep it from working at peak capacity include eating too much refined sugar and refined carbohydrates and greasy foods, as well as excessive worrying. Another major culprit: worrying or "thinking too much." This is believed to can clog up our energies, causing a disharmony between the spleen (thinking) and the heart (spirit). Sometimes, something as simple as changing your diet and exercising more to help clear your head and work off excess energies is all that is needed to realign the spleen with the other organs that may have impeded conception in the past.

The Liver and Gallbladder

The Chinese believe that the liver is directly responsible for ovulation since it also handles blood filtration, blood flow and the metabolism of hormones throughout the body.

Right before a woman menstruates, her liver begins to redirect blood flow from other bodily organs to the uterus. Creating this back-up of Qi energy outside of the uterus is what causes those monthly cramps, headaches, sadness, and more.

The fact is, if the liver and gallbladder are not functioning properly or become blocked, the hormone releases related to reproduction could be impeded. If the Qi is left to stagnate in the liver, the uterus will in turn become a hostile place for a fertilized egg, causing an implantation failure or even a miscarriage.

The Uterus

The Chinese call the uterus "the palace for the child." Although it is an independent organ, it is very sensitive to any disturbance within the rest of the body. Should any connection between it and the rest of the body become blocked or cut, conception cannot occur.

How Chinese Medicine Can Help You Achieve Your Conception Goals

If a woman is to conceive, according to Traditional Chinese Medicine, her reproductive organs must stay in alignment with the rest of her body's organs (and energy).   There are many things which can disrupt the flow of natural energies including stress, chemicals, and a lack of exercise, poor eating, excessive emotions and more.   Even a slight aberration can throw off the entire system, making it harder to get pregnant. Considering all of the things which can create chaos amongst the body's energies, it may seem impossible to deal with these negative influences; but it isn't. The body easily responds to gentle persuasion toward balance: and that's what Chinese medicine is all about.

Eastern Medicine believes that there is always a reason that part of your body is not working properly, and once the disturbance is discovered it can be treated in order to restore balance and alleviate symptoms – including infertility.

The key to finding the imbalances in your own body that could be impeding your ability to have children is to be evaluated by a trained professional in Traditional Chinese Medicine.   Once the source of your Qi disruption has been discovered he can prescribe a treatment regimen that is guaranteed to work to heal your specific problems and symptoms.

What Western Medicine Has to Say About Infertility – and Why They're Often Wrong

American couples spend more than $2 billion a year on fertility treatments, according to recent reports. Yet, more than half of them still fail to conceive.

With dozens of high-tech procedures at our disposal, you'd think that anyone – and everyone – who wanted to get pregnant could – and would. Still, many do not. Why? More often than not it is because modern medical practitioners fail to do what Eastern practitioners do: look for the most subtle things which could impede conception that have little or nothing to do with a health problem.

True, IVF or other such medical procedures can help fertilize an egg via a Petrie dish and bypass any blockages within the woman's reproductive system, but if her emotions and inner energies are not considered (and treated), implantation will not – and often cannot – occur.

The biggest problem with western medicine, according to those who prescribe to a more Eastern worldview, is their need to find and "fix" a conception problem with a pill or a procedure instead of finding ways to help the body heal itself more naturally. Here's an example: let's say your thyroid is not producing the proper amounts of the hormone needed for pregnancy, western medicine dictates prescribing a synthetic hormone to fix the imbalance; while eastern medicine looks for reasons why the thyroid isn't working properly and finds a treatment that will help coax the thyroid into making proper amounts of the needed hormone on its own again.

Of course that doesn't mean that modern technology should never be used to treat infertility; only that it should be used in conjunction with other methods designed to bring the entire body into alignment in order to guarantee success. For many women a combination of western and eastern treatment methods is the best course of action in helping them conceive.

Chinese Medicine – Infertility Questionnaire

It doesn't matter whether you rely on Western medicine; Eastern medicine or a combination of both to solve your conception issues if you don't have a clear diagnosis of your problem. Of course, the path you take toward finding the right diagnosis depends a great deal on which worldview you prescribe in. Western medicine relies on scientific and often invasive tests and procedures to discover what is wrong; while Eastern medicine relies on observing a patient's color, breathing patterns, movements, tongue and so on, as well as finding the three pulse locations and observing changes in each, as a way to evaluate symptoms and discover why you may be having a hard time getting pregnant. For most patients, that requires filling out an intensive questionnaire designed to give the practitioner a good hard look at every aspect of her health and lifestyle.

When it comes to fertility issues, eastern medical practitioners look at the four organ systems (kidney, spleen, heart and liver) and the Yin, Yang, Qi and Blood for disruptions. Finding out which diagnostic category a woman falls under is important to determining the proper course of action. In order to have a better idea of what system failure may be causing your infertility issues, answer the questions below. One important one here: it is very rare that only one disruption is present, so some of your answers may overlap, steering your practitioner toward several problem areas. That's perfectly normal and should be expected.

Keep in mind that this questionnaire is not meant to help you self-diagnose your own problems, but to give you a better idea of what may be keeping you from having the baby you so badly want. Once you have a better idea of what may inhibiting your ability to conceive, you can look for a practitioner experienced in battling just those types of problems.

Answer yes or no to the questions in each diagnostic category. If you find yourself answering yes to more than one-quarter of the questions, note that category and be sure to let your health care provider know as well as your TCM specialist. In addition to that, within the 5-Step Natural Pregnancy chapter we would discuss exactly how to tackle your unique energy disorder using the powers of traditional Chinese medicine including herbal, nutritional and lifestyle recommendations.

Kidney Yin Deficiency

Do you have a history of knee pain or disorders?

Do you suffer from tinnitus (hissing, ringing or buzzing sounds in your ears)?

Are you often restlessness?

Do you have difficulty getting good-quality sleep?

Are you flushing easily?

Do you frequently in need of drinking fluids?

Is your period flow scanty?

Do you experience heavy bright-red periods?

In your BBT- is the follicular phase often unsteady or longer than the usual 13 or 14 days?

Is your pulse weak or gives the impression of "floating" under the skin?

Is your tongue dry and small?

Is your tongue red with little coat?

Do you often experience dizziness?

Do you often feel anxious or afraid?

Do you suffer from vaginal dryness?

Do you often experience lower back pain or weakness?

Do you have dark spots or circles under your eyes?

Are you relatively young and still have too much gray hair?

Kidney Yang Deficiency

Are you overweight or feel puffed?

Do you often experience lethargy?

Do you have low motivation?

Do you experience pain in the knees and legs?

Do you experience diarrhea before the beginning of the period?

Do you have clots in the menstrual flow?

In your BBT chart, are the readings quite low(36.0°C or 96.8°F or less)

Is your pulse slow and deep?

Is your tongue pale and swollen?

Is your urine diluted?

Is your lower back often feels weak or sore?

Are your hands and feet often cold?

Do you often have more sensitivity to cold than those around you?

Prior to your period, do you often experience pain in your lower back?

Do you experience loose stools and even urgent stools early in the morning?

Do you experience low libido?

Is your menses dull in color?

Do you find yourself waking once or more during the night to urinate?

Do you urinate frequently?

Do you frequently experience vaginal discharge?

Heart Qi Stagnation

Is the tip of your tongue red?

Do you often experience nightmares?

Do you often feel agitated or edgy?

Do you fidget?

Do you often having troubles sleeping after waking up early in the morning?

Do you often experience palpitations?

Do you often experience anxiety?

Do you often experience insomnia?

Do you experience extreme neurosis?

Were you diagnosed with a pituitary gland which under or over-producing

FSH or LH?

Are your estrogen levels low?

In your BBT chart, in the follicular phase do you see high peaks or a very

unsteady graph?

Is your pulse choppy or tight feeling?

Do you sweat a lot?

Blood Qi Stagnation

Can you observe clots and tissue in the menstrual flow?

Is your menstrual flow incomplete, clotty or unsmooth?

Do you suffer from hair loss?

Is your skin dry?

Do you have acne on your face?

In your BBT chart, does the temperature not fall to its low level immediately when the new cycle starts?
.

Are your menses late?

Does your pulse feel tight when there is pain?

Does your tongue have a purplish hue or show some purple areas?

Phlegm-Damp Accumulation

Do you suffer from pituitary tumors, ovarian cysts or endometrial congestion?

Do you suffer from acne?

Does your stool have bright and foul-smell

Are you overeating rich, sweet food often?

Are you feeling tired most of the day?

Are you obese or have a tendency to put on weight?

Are your menstrual periods often scanty and thick or mucusy?

Do you suffer from joint ache?

Do you experience irregularly spaced menses?

Do you experience vaginal discharges?

Is your tongue often coated with a thick or greasy coat?

Spleen Qi Deficiency

Is your nose often cold?

Do you have low blood pressure?

Is your complexion yellowish or pale?

Do you feel bloated after a meal?

Are your hands and feet often cold?

Do you often feel sluggish or fatigue?

Do you often feel no desire to eat?

Do you find yourself bruised or sick easily?

Are you often constipated?

Do you have varicose veins?

Do you experience cravings for refined carbohydrates?

Are your stools loose?

Do you often have digestion problems such as stomach cramps, gas, heartburn?

Are your arms and legs weak?

Is your menses thin, watery, or pinkish in color?

Do you suffer from a wide range of allergies?

Do you have a history of anemia? (Even one occasion)

Do you have a history of uterine prolapse? (Even one occasion)

Do you suffer from hemorrhoids?

Do you sweat a lot, even without exerting yourself?

Do you feel dizzy or lightheaded if you stand up too quickly?

Liver Qi Stagnation

Right before your period, do you often feel irritable?

Upon ovulation, do you experience digestion problems such as bloating?

Do you often feel depressed?

Do you often feel intense irritability to the point of uncontrollable anger?

Do you experience headaches with bloodshot eyes?

In your BBT chart, in the earlier parts of the cycle do you see instability or temperature peaks?

Is your pulse wiry?

Do you experience significantly long ovulation periods?

Do you experience mild to severe insomnia?

Upon waking up, do you often feel a sour taste in your mouth?

Do you experience painful, thick or dark periods?

Is your tongue dark or purplish in color?

Do you often suffer from acid reflux?

Upon ovulation, are your breasts feel tender or in pain?

Do you experience discharge from your nipples or pain in that area?

Have you been diagnosed with elevated prolactin levels?

Are your pupils dilated and large?

Now that you have a clearer picture of what energy deficiencies could be stopping conception, it's time to find a qualified Chinese Medical practitioner for help. Within the 5-Step Natural Pregnancy chapter we would discuss exactly how to address each of these deficiencies using the powers of traditional Chinese medicine including herbal, nutritional and lifestyle recommendations.

Chapter Four

The 5-Step Plan for Getting Pregnant and Having Healthy Babies

Introduction

Chinese medicine hinges on an ancient philosophy called the Tao, which looks at everything in the universe (including fertility) as an interaction between opposites: hot and cold; light and dark; male and female; and so on. The Chinese describe these opposite energies as the Yin and the Yang. According to Chinese beliefs, the Yin and Yang are present in every living thing, with each energy having a small part of the other hidden away inside of it. For example, the shortest day of the year is also the point where the days begin to grow longer. See how each day contains a large part of one energy source and a smaller part of the other?

To describe the Yin and the Yang, the Chinese like to use examples from nature. For instance, the Yin is usually thought of like water (yielding, receiving, cold, slow, passive and heavy); while the Yang is considered like fire (hot, quick, bright and aggressive). Maybe that's why the Yin is considered more female, while the Yang is considered to have more male qualities.

Keep in mind, however, that not every woman is (or should be) all Yin, and every man all Yang. Chinese philosophy looks for balance between the two energies in everything. In order for the body to work properly, it must contain some portion of its opposite energy. This is called mutual restraint and is considered a must for optimal health.

Let's take a quick look at how an imbalance of a woman's Yin and Yang energies can affect her fertility. Estrogen (Yin energy) is a dominant hormone when it comes to fertility. It is what creates the uterine lining needed to nourish a fetus and even prepares the passageway for the sperm to reach the uterus for fertilization.

As a woman approaches menopause, her estrogen levels (or Yin energies) drop, causing hot flashes, night sweats and vaginal dryness. The hotter Yang energy begins to take over.

It is your Yang energy which invigorates your reproductive system and tells it to produces testosterone and progesterone, two hormones needed (in the proper amounts) to transform the endometrial tissues so it can hold a fertilized egg.

Your thyroid also expels Yang energy. That's why people with overactive thyroids often feel anxious, hot, and may experience insomnia; while people without enough thyroid action (insufficient heat sensations form the Yang); are always cold and tired.

Without the right amounts of both Yin and Yang energies (estrogen progesterone, testosterone and thyroid secretions), the reproductive organs can not do their jobs properly. And this could cause an inability to get pregnant.

So, what can you do to make sure that your Yin and Yang are in balance? Here are five ways every woman can help to strengthen her reproductive system naturally using Traditional Chinese Medicine techniques:

Step One: Achieving Balance, Harmony and Congruency for Conceiving Your Baby

Thus far, you have learned a lot about your menstrual cycles and the ways in which your body prepares for creating and nourishing new life within the womb. All of this information can leave you feeling a bit overwhelmed. Don't be. While it is important to understand how your body works, you can easily divide your menstrual cycle into two main phases for the purposes of getting and staying pregnant.

The Two-Phase Approach for Achieving Balance and Harmony and Creating the Perfect Environment for Conceiving a Baby

From now on, when you think of your cycle, divide it into these two simple phases:

Before Ovulation

After Ovulation

It doesn't really matter whether you have ovulated or not; or whether you are pregnant or not. Right now your job is to prepare your body for conception and then for the job ahead of caring for your growing baby.

Phase I: Before Ovulation begins with the first day of your menstrual flow and continues until you ovulate. This is an important time of preparing your body for conception. It includes giving your body the rest, relaxation and nourishment it needs to get ready to make a baby! It is important during Phase I of your cycle to create a calm, stable internal environment for your egg and your partner's sperm to join together in life. This is not a time for excitement, stress or even increases in your heart rate or circulation. Instead, opt for quiet, calm activities and do your best to keep your body in harmony.

Phase II: After Ovulation, can either be a time of rest for your body (if you are not pregnant); or a time of work (if you are pregnant). Your body has to be ready for either scenario, and this requires taking extra precautions in all areas of your life to ensure that if conception has occurred, you are giving that embryo every chance to implant and survive. Again, calm is the key here. Avoid any strenuous activities including exercises or lovemaking that may cause cramping, abdominal stimulation or an activation of the muscles in the pelvic floor. This includes sit-ups, walking up and down stairs, doing Kegels or even enjoying vigorous lovemaking.

To ensure that your body is creating the proper environment for a pregnancy, be sure to avoid these activities 24 hours prior to ovulation until your period begins:

Air travel – there are a lot of things about air travel that can disrupt your energy Qi: the stress of travelling; air pressure changes; and more. At a time when you need to keep your internal weather calm, flying can cause some real turbulence to your fertility energies.

Bumpy bus or car rides – not only are bumpy train, bus or car rides stressful emotionally, but they can also be stressful physically, putting undo (and maybe even dangerous) pressure on the reproductive organs and/or pelvic region.

Emotional Upheaval. Avoid anyone or anything that you might find
emotionally upsetting can disrupt your ability to both conceive and to aid the implantation of a fertilized embryo. Remember, anything that effects your body's internal Qi will affect your fertility.

Hot baths. If there is one thing that you do not want to do when you are
trying to get pregnant is to increase your body heat. Hot baths and saunas do just that. While they may feel relaxing externally, internally hot baths will raise your internal temperature, thus disrupting your internal Qi.

Aromatherapy can be a strong form of treatment for certain disorders.
Fertility, however, often responds negatively to strong pungent odors from bath oils, incense, essential oils and even candles. These types of scented products can dramatically affect the way the blood and Qi energy flow through the body, which may inhibit pregnancy in some women.

Ginger While it may be used to ease morning sickness, ginger and ginger
products can actually disperse energy within the body, causing improper blood flow which can prevent a pregnancy form either occurring or thriving.

The 8 Commandments of This Program

It isn't enough to follow the rules listed above, you must commit to following these 8 basic commandments of the program if you want to increase your chances of getting (and staying) pregnant:

Commandment # 1: Get plenty of rest. Make a decision to go to bed

early and get up later. Your body needs at least 8 hours of good quality sleep in order to be able to withstand the rigors of a pregnancy.

Commandment # 2: Stop eating Junk food. Now is not the time to fill

your body with a lot of sugar, additives and preservatives. Give your body the nutrients it needs to do the job you have in store for it. Fill up on plenty of fresh foods including vegetables and whole grains.

Commandment # 3: Exercise regularly. If only to walk around the

block at lunchtime, be sure to get some sort of physical exercise each and every day.

Commandment # 4: Stop Smoking. It's horrible for you – and worse

for a growing fetus!

Commandment # 5: Stay Away from alcohol and caffeine. That

means no more sugared drinks, soda pop, coffee and cocktails.

| Page 105

Commandment # 6: Stay away from cold foods and drinks. Don't add ice to your drinks or indulge in freezer foods like ice cream.

Commandment #7: Wear a hat. Be sure to dress warmly in the colder months and be sure to keep your head covered in all sorts of weather.

Commandment #8: Be sure to dry your hair before stepping outdoors. Never leave the house with a wet head.

Step Two: Using Diet, Vitamins & Minerals to Enhance Fertility

Diet and lifestyle can have a direct impact on your ability to conceive. How? Eat the wrong foods, or participate in the wrong habits and your immune system can be compromised. Without a healthy immune system your organs can't perform properly and your blood can't flow the way it should. This can all create an imbalance in your body that prohibits one of its most important jobs: conceiving and nurturing a baby.

It doesn't matter whether you follow traditional western medicine or a more eastern philosophy to tackle your infertility issues, taking better care of your body is always a good idea when you are trying to conceive. After all, if you don't give your body the proper mix of vitamins and minerals, how can you expect it to handle such a complicated (and important) job as creating another living being.

So, where should you start when trying to improve your overall health? Let's begin with the basics: what you eat:

Dietary Guidelines: Eating for Two

We've all heard pregnant women say "I'm eating for two," as they pile the food on their plate. The fact is you should begin eating for two long before a baby is ever growing inside of you. Now, I don't mean adding 2,000 extra calories to your diet. I mean, learning to eat in a way that makes your body strong and able to work at peak efficiency. If you don't eat properly, your hormones could be thrown out of whack; your organs will fail to work in unison the way they need to; and you'll find it easier to get pregnant. Not that diet can fix any infertility problem, but it sure is a good place to start.

Food is the source of all energy. But, did you know that different types of foods have their own quality of energy? Well, they do! Too much (or too little) of certain vitamins and mineral containing nutrients and your body won't be balanced. This imbalance can restrict its ability to work the way it should and could affect your fertility.

According to Chinese medical philosophies, the Shen (or kidney and spirit) oversee a woman's the reproductive system. While you are looking at the many reasons why you can't get pregnant, you may want to consider boosting your Shen with an intake foods like walnuts, black sesame seeds, barley, tofu, soybean, wheat germ and seaweeds.

So, what dietary changes should you consider when trying to conceive? Here are a few all women should adhere to (no matter what their fertility obstacle):

Get Plenty of Fatty Acids

Every living cell in your body requires sufficient amounts of linoleic acid and alpha-linoleic acid to stay healthy. They are also a key to ovulation, so eating plenty of fish, fish oil, soy, eggs, broccoli, and dark green vegetables can all help prepare your body for the job ahead.

One Important Note Here: while eating fish is a great way to get essential fatty acids in your diet, pregnant women (and those who are trying to get pregnant) need to avoid fish that are at the top of the food chain (shark, flake, tuna, etc). High levels of mercury are often found in these fish and the higher you go on the food chain, the more mercury is found. Not sure which fish to avoid; use this simple rule: stay away from fish that eat other fish to survive.

Scale Back on Acidic Foods

An uneven PH level in your reproductive system can inhibit conception, so be sure to eat plenty of non-citrus fruits, vegetables, sprouts, cereal grasses and herbs to even out those Ph levels.

Eat Plenty of Cruciferous Vegetables

Cruciferous vegetables like cabbage, cauliflower, broccoli and Brussels sprouts all contain the compound Di-indolylmethane (DIM), which is known to increase the metabolism of Estradiol (a form of Estrogen) in the body.

Eat Only Organic and Hormone Free Meats

The foods we eat aren't always good for us – even if it isn't considered "junk food." For some women, the pesticides, chemicals and hormones found in today's meats can also interfere with natural hormone production and cause infertility.

Every time you eat something that has an additive, preservative or artificial flavor, you are not only robbing your body of the chance to get the right nutrients from that particular food, but you are stripping your body of the nutrients it has already collected. How? When you add these elements to your body, it is forced to use valuable nutrients to detoxify it.

Avoid Refined Carbohydrates

Our bodies take the essential vitamins and minerals in the foods we eat and uses them to metabolize everything we eat. Unfortunately, when whole grains are refined, many of these important minerals are stripped away. If you eat too many refined carbohydrates like white bread, plain pasta and white rice, your body may be forced to tap into its mineral stores to get what it needs. This can oftentimes result in a zinc or folic acid deficiency in your body. This can be detrimental to a pregnancy and fetus. Sufficient levels of zinc are essential to increase sperm counts in men and too little zinc in either parent's body can result in chromosomal abnormalities, and fetal death. A Folic acid deficiency can result in reduced production of eggs and sperm, as well as spina bifida if babies.

Avoid Dairy Products

Most dairy products these days contain high levels of hormones used to encourage the cows to produce more milk, as well as pesticides used in the feed they are given. Ingesting these hormones can cause your own levels to become altered and also corrupt a growing fetus.

Dairy products (especially cow's milk) cause allergies, create heavy mucus, and clog your digestive tracts. Dairy products are loaded with hormones injected to the animals in order to increase their capacity to produce milk. Dairy products are filled with antibiotics, which is destructive to your body and hormonal balance.
In fact, humans are the only species that drink the milk of other species. The problem is that we cannot digest the milk as calves do. Our digestion system is built differently. We cannot process the protein in milk either. This often leads to multiple types of allergic reactions, mucus buildup and digestion problems that manifest themselves as candida yeast infection and reproductive disorders.

What to avoid: milk and cheese, products that have lactose, milk proteins, whey protein and dry skim milk powder.

Good substitutes: sesame seed butter. This is ground whole sesame seeds (not the regular Tahini), a wonderful source of protein and calcium containing more than 1100 mg of calcium per 100 g.

Good alternatives to dairy products also include nut/seed milks (sesame seeds, almonds, pumpkin seeds etc. excluding cashews and peanuts).

Soy products can also serve as an alternative but should be consumed sparingly because excessive consumption has been linked to thyroid problems.

Eliminate Caffeine, Nicotine and Alcohol From Your Diet

All stimulants should be avoided when trying to conceive. Nicotine can age your ovaries and make your eggs resistant to fertilization, especially as you age; alcohol is extremely harmful to fertility, with western researchers reporting a 50% decrease in the success of treatment for women undergoing IVF who had consumed even minimal amounts of alcohol; and caffeine can restrict blood vessels in both men and women, causing fertility problems.

Avoid All Unnecessary Medications and Over the Counter Drugs

Unless absolutely necessary, all medications should be stopped while trying to get pregnant since they can affect every organ of the body and the energy they emit.

Avoid Junk Food

Giving your body too much sugar, carbohydrates and an overabundance of other unhealthy foods can all contribute to infertility by not providing the right nutrition necessary to keep your body in its best and healthiest shape. For instance, eating too many saturated fats can interfere with the metabolism of those essential fatty acids you need, which can create a hormonal imbalance.

Note About Fruit

We have talked a bit about the negative impact refined sugars can have on your health and fertility. That does not mean that you should necessarily avoid eating fruit. Sweet by nature, many fruits offer a wonderfully healthy way to get the vitamins and minerals you need, as well as a way to get a sweet sugar fix. Eating a baked apple with honey can be a real appetite pleaser, as well as a friendly fertility food to indulge in once in awhile.

Fresh fruit can also benefit your fertility by help to calm your body – something refined sugars can't (and don't) do. There are some exceptions though. For instance, if you are internally very cool, you will want to stay away from all raw foods – including fresh fruits.

No matter what your internal temperature, it is always a good idea to stay away from both hot-energy and cold-energy fruits like pineapple, mangos and melons when trying to get pregnant. Choose instead such energy neutral fruits as raspberries, grapes, apples and pears. This will help to ensure that the food you eat isn't disrupting your body's harmony.

Note About Raw Food

It would make sense that raw foods are better for you. Right? Not necessarily; especially if you are trying to get pregnant. Digesting raw foods takes a lot of energy – more so than digesting cooked (warm) foods. Now, if you happen to be one of those women with a cooler constitution, digesting those cool raw foods can sap your body of the Qi energy it needs to accept and sustain a pregnancy. This is especially true during colder weather. So, if you know you have a cooler constitution and are finding it difficult to get pregnant, stay away from raw foods of any kind. Heat up all foods, or at least keep them at room temperature. This should help boost your Qi energy, helping to give your body the support it needs to make your baby.

Supplementation to Enhance Fertility

To help you achieve successful conception, make sure you have the right amounts of these important vitamins and minerals either through your diet and/or supplements:

Essential Fatty Acids (EFA)

One of the main causes of hormonal imbalance in the human body is an insufficient level of prostaglandins, which are chemicals that help regulate hormones as they communicate between hormones and human cells. The more hormones your body produces (during menstruation, for example), the more it needs prostaglandins to stabilize and regulate these hormones. The only problem is that the body cannot manufacture sufficient amounts of prostaglandins without the proper raw materials.

These raw materials are the **essential fatty acids (EFA).**

EFAs also support the immune and nervous system.

EFAs are found in flax oil, cold water fish such as salmon or tuna, sunflower seeds, soybean, borage, walnut and safflower oil.

Omega-3, omega-6, and omega-9 are the essential fatty acids your body needs to produce the critical prostaglandins. However, it's not enough that you consume foods rich in EFA like salmon and flax oil and walnuts. You need to have the proper balance of these EFAs in order for your body to effectively produce these prostaglandins.

Because a typical western diet (even a healthy diet) is rich in omega-6 and omega-9 (olive oil, canola oil) but poor in omega-3, you'll obviously need to balance your EFA intake by consuming more cold fish oil, walnuts and flax oil that are rich in omega-3. The recommended ratio is twice the amount of omega-3 than omega-6 and omega-9 combined.

Taking EFA supplements will ensure your body has all the raw materials it needs to produce the necessary prostaglandins to stabilize your hormones.

EFAs will also help control excess insulin production (Recent studies show a strong link between fatty acid composition and insulin action).

The only one I recommend, having experienced it myself, is the Total EFA-Vegetarian Formula (a liquid). It is an excellent source of EFA. The magic 3 oils (flax, borage and primrose) are cold-processed, organic and kept in a dark bottle unexposed to oxygen, heat or sunlight.

Recommended amount per day: 2 to 4 tablespoons.

Important: The **Total EFA** comes in a gel cap formula and a liquid vegetarian formula. Be sure to buy the liquid formula as it is far superior. Also, be sure to keep the bottle refrigerated at all times.

Available at: **http://www.bodybuilding.com/store/sun/efa.html**

NAC (N-Acetyl Cysteine)

NAC (N-Acetyl Cysteine) maintains the proper functioning of the lungs and supports the immune system and liver function. NAC is also a powerful antioxidant. It acts as mucolytic and increases levels of glutathione in the body. It can also be useful for insulin resistance and improving fertility.

A recent study shows that NAC dramatically reduced testosterone levels and homocysteine levels and had a significant positive impact on insulin secretion and insulin resistance in 6 lean and 31 obese women with PCOS who participated in the study.

Available from:

http://www.amazon.com/Nac

Vitamin A

Vitamin A helps the body produce the proper amounts of cervical mucus in women, and protect sperm in males from damaging free radicals. A deficiency in Vitamin A is shown to reduce sperm volume and count, and increase abnormal sperm so it is suggested that both men and women get up to 10,000 IU of Beta Carotene. The best foods to eat for this purpose include: carrots, sweet potatoes, cantaloupe, spinach, eggs, yellow fruits and vegetables, whole milk and milk products, dark green leafy veggies, and fish oils.

B Vitamins

Women can benefit from B6 as a way to keep your ovaries healthy and working well. Suggested **Dosage**: B6: 50mg - 100mg per day; B12: 1000 mcg per day; B-complex: contains 50mcg B12, 50mg all other B vitamins. B Vitamins can be found in the following foods: beans, nuts, legumes, eggs, meats, fish and whole grains

d-Pinitol 600

d-Pinitol is a naturally occurring compound that can be found in foods. Certain natural substances can be beneficial to support and maintain ovarian health in women. Potentially effective approaches include dietary modifications designed to improve insulin sensitivity and supplementation with D-chiro-inositol (or d-pinitol), vitamin D, and chromium. Regular use of these strategies can help promote, improve, and support ovarian health and insulin sensitivity, resulting in overall positive health benefits.

In one study, D-chiro-inositol was given to 44 obese women with PCOS (1,200 mg once a day) or placebo for eight weeks. The D-chiro-inositol group had ovulated more, showed a dramatic improvement in insulin resistance, and had a 55% reduction in testosterone levels compared to the placebo group.

Suggested Dosage: 1–2 capsules twice daily with meals.

Available from:

http://www.drhoffman.com

Vitex 750 - Chaste Tree Extract

VITEX 750 contains a high dose Vitex extract that is fortified with Vitex essential oil making it a powerful clinical tool to support women during times of hormonal change. Vitex helps maintain healthy prolactin and hormonal balance during the monthly menstrual cycle. Vitex helps support breast comfort and a normal healthy attitude and mood during the menstrual cycle. Vitex also helps maintain normal ovarian function, trigger the production of progesterone and helps women with lack of ovulation or infertility.

Available from:

http://www.vitaminmegashop.com/product.php?productid=16596

Cinnulin PF (Highly Recommended)

Cinnulin PF® is the only patented aqueous cinnamon extract available and is manufactured through an innovative water-based process using no chemical solvents. Cinnulin PF is produced from a superior source of cinnamon bark, validated to have the highest concentration of active Type-A Polymers that have been shown to support healthy blood sugar metabolism and cholesterol management, weight management and displays potent antioxidant properties.

Recent studies showed that the consumption of cinnamon reduced insulin resistance in fifteen PCOS women and women with infertility issues.

Not to be taken by pregnant or lactating women.

Available from:

http://www.vitaminmegashop.com

Vitamin C

A powerful antioxidant that protects the essential fatty acids, vitamin C also helps with male infertility (sperm motility), speeds up the healing process and enhances thymus function. It also neutralizes toxins and reduces stress.

Vitamin C is naturally found in red bell peppers, oranges, lemons, watermelons, kiwi, strawberries, green leafy vegetables, broccoli and parsley.

You can provide yourself with vitamin C simply by eating organic citrus fruit or strawberries in the morning. Squeezing organic lemon juice and diluting it with water cannot only provide a high quality of vitamin C, it also cleanses your system when taken on an empty stomach.

The recommended amount per day is 1000 mg.

Available at: **http://www.amazon.com/VitaminC**

Vitamin E

One of the most powerful antioxidants available, protecting the body from free radicals and preventing polyunsaturated fats from becoming oxidized, vitamin E helps with infertility issues both with men and women, repairs skin damage, speeds up the healing process and enhances thymus function.

Naturally found in avocadoes, carrots, celery, leek, lettuce, parsnip sweet potatoes, Brussels sprouts, cabbage and spinach, whole wheat flour, whole wheat bran, whole grain cereals, oatmeal, soy beans, legumes, raw unadulterated honey, bee pollen, sprouted seeds and sweet potatoes.

The recommended daily amount is at least 400 IU in the form of natural, dry d-alpha tocopherol.

Available at: **http://www.amazon.com/VitaminE**

Borage Oil

Adding extra amount of Borage oil to the Total EFA blend, to ensure proper GLA intake and the production of anti-inflammatory hormones, has yielded tremendously positive results with some PCOS women especially among women who have infertility issues/ovarian cysts or go through painful PMS symptoms.

You can find Borage Liquid Gold by Health From the Sun's at: **http://www.vitacost.com/**

Colostrum

Colostrum is one of the best and most effective supplements to support the immune system. With the help of 36 different immune elements, colostrum boosts and regulates the immune system and fights infections in the gut like no other supplement available.

Lactoferrin, found in Immunecare Colostrum, has great anti-bacterial, antifungal and anti-viral properties.

Colostrum has been found to be very effective at autoimmune disorders typical among women with infertility issues.

Colostrum is available from **http://www.immunecare.co.uk/**.

Note: if you are lactose intolerant you can try the other brand:

http://immunecare.co.uk/product1.html - LACTASE

The above product contains both lactase and protease enzymes, which help break down the lactose in milk and thus prevent the typical problems associated with dairy consumption.

Q-10 Supplement

Coenzyme (Q-10) supplements are a great way to improve cellular function and decrease any decline in egg quality that may be experienced with age. Traditionally used to treat cardiovascular disorders, Q-10 is considered the "powerhouse" of the cell and is also linked to repairing free radical cell damage which can prevent pregnancy and inhibit implantation.

As you can see, there are plenty of vitamins and minerals that can enhance reproduction and keep your reproductive organs healthy. In addition, there are several natural supplements that can help restore a natural balance of these minerals in your body including:

Bee pollen and Royal Jelly -- is said to alleviate menstrual problems in women and increase sperm production in men

Blue-Green Algae – great for the immune system it is said to regulate metabolism, repair damaged tissues and tonify Qi energy and the blood.

Wheatgrass – used to nourish the Qi, blood and essence, while enhancing immunity and restoring hormonal balance.

Vitamin B6 – it helps the body metabolize excess energy; produce the right amounts of progesterone and restore imbalanced periods.

Folic Acid – important in cellular division, higher doses of folic acid are recommended to alleviate many birth defects.

Take a Multi-vitamin and Mineral Complex

If your body is missing certain vitamins it can affect your hormone levels and even impede your ability to become pregnant. Using a variety of vitamin supplements and minerals can help balance your hormone levels, as well as your spouse's and increase your chances of having a baby.   The first place to begin is by taking a good multi-vitamin or prenatal vitamin (for women).

Eliminate Toxins

Some researchers estimate that our bodies are bombarded with up to 300 different chemicals each and every day. No wonder we are experiencing health effects of all of this abuse! No matter how well you eat and how carefully you control your environment, everyone is bombarded with dozens of toxins everyday – and some of them may be the root cause of your infertility! From air pollution, cleaning products, garden sprays, and even radiation from our cell phones and building materials, our bodies are under constant attack. And it is fighting back. While it may be possible to take some of these toxins out of your environment, some have to be dealt with in another way to reverse their effects: through supplementation. Here are the major areas of concern to investigate for toxins in your life:

Water

It isn't just the water you drink that could be a problem, The water you take a bath and shower in can also seep into your system through the skin, causing concern. Your first step to making sure the water you come in contact with is safe is to install a high quality water purification system in your home to remove chemicals, pesticides, herbicides, insecticides, lead, allergens, Giardia and cryptosporidium from the water you drink, cook with and bathe with. Also, consider installing a filter on your shower for even more protection, since hot water can make many toxins more volatile and more easily absorbed.

Lead

Lead can be very dangerous to your nervous system and is often found in older homes built or remodeled prior to the 1970's. There are simple home tests you can purchase to see if any lead resides in your home, or you can hire a professional lead-finder to do a more detailed search.

Mercury

Almost everyone comes in contact with mercury on a regular basis. It is found in many common household items (electrical components, pesticides and some cosmetics), as well as some of the fish we eat (tuna and shark). One controversial source of mercury is amalgam fillings, which some believe may begin to leach after a few years. If you suspect that high mercury levels may be causing your infertility, have your levels checked by a kinesiologist, a diagnostic process which uses "muscle tests" to identify a problem.

Cleaning products

There are plenty of cleaning products on the market that should be avoided by everyone – but especially couples trying to conceive. Luckily, green products are easy to find these days and offer a toxin-free way to keep your home clean and tidy.

Gardening products

Lawn and garden sprays can all present a hazard to couples trying to conceive. Forget the pesticides for a more natural lawn and garden.

Environmental Toxins

Our environment is riddled with toxins that may be prohibiting our ability to procreate. Some of the biggest culprits include xenohormones (petro-chemically derived pesticides, emulsifiers found in soap and cosmetics, plastics and regular meat). These types of man-made chemicals which can be found in our food and environment, can cause hormone dysfunction, ovary damage (damaged follicles which cause reduced production of progesterone) and other infertility problems.

Solvents are the most common type of xenohormones we are exposed to on a regular basis and are usually found in glue, dry cleaning clothes, nail polish and paint. They can lead to an array of health problems including fatigue, anxiety, depression, brain swelling, and fetus damage and oxygen deprivation in the brain.

Worse yet (when trying to conceive), these xenohormones tend to mimic estrogen activity in the body, causing hormonal imbalances by damaging the ovaries that results in low progesterone levels, activating estrogen receptor sites, and by hindering the ability of the liver to produce estrogen. This can eventually lead to the development of ovarian cysts, which can further impede your chance of becoming parents.

The exposure of female embryos to xenobiotics (environmental pollutants that mimic the chemical activity of estrogen on the developing baby's tissues), damage the female ovarian follicles and make them dysfunctional. They are then unable to complete ovulation or produce sufficient progesterone.

Sound scary? Well, it is! I can't stress enough the importance of minimizing your exposure to these environmental chemicals.

Here are some guidelines for decreasing your exposure to these destructive toxic chemicals:

1. Eat only organically grown or cared for foods

2. Avoid fabric softeners, air fresheners, plastic clothing, plastic storage or heating using plastics.

3. Don't use pesticides or house sprays for bugs, pets or for your lawn or garden.

4. Install an air purifier for cleaner air

5. Use only non-toxic "green" paint

6. Install stone or tile in your home. The glue found in most carpets releases toxic molecules on a daily basis.

7. Cleanse and detoxify your bowels, kidneys and liver every 2-3 months.

Nutritional and Lifestyle Suggestions to Treat Your Individual Problem According To TCM

As you've learned, there are a lot of ways to enhance your ability to get pregnant simply by eating foods designed to help fix any deficiencies your body may be experiencing. Below you will find a myriad of diet and lifestyle suggestions to guide you through a variety of diagnostic conditions:

Kidney Yin Deficiency

Eat plenty of:

wheat germ

barley

rice

asparagus

black beans

kidney beans

red beans

string beans

chick peas

Brussels sprouts

beets

apples, bananas, raspberries, blackberries, grapes, lemons, pineapple, mangoes

and mulberries

shellfish

eggs

organ meats not treated with hormones

soy and flaxseed

Avoid dry pungent spices such as pepper, curry, and horseradish.

Avoid over exercising.

Avoid saunas.

Do not participate in Bikram Yoga.

Kidney Yang Deficiency

Follow the dietary suggestions for Kidney Essence Deficiency

Eat lots of warm, nourishing foods

Eat at least three servings of hormone free meat or animal products per day

Eat plenty of lentils, gingerroot and black beans

Eat plenty of oats, grains, sweet brown rice and quinoa

Eat walnuts regularly

Eat Yang-type vegetables (winter squash, cabbage, kale, leeks, chives, parsley, garlic and scallions)

Cook with peppers and other warming spices

Take warm baths regularly

Use a heating pad on your feet and lower abdomen

exercise moderately

Use L-Arginine supplements

Kidney Deficiency (both Yin and Yang)

Eat the following foods as much as possible:

black beans

legumes

kelp

parsley

wheat germ/wheat grass

string beans

mulberry

millet

organ meats (not treated with hormones)

tonify

oysters, clams, lobster

raspberries

walnuts

chestnuts

black sesame seeds

yams

gelatin

corn

Avoid all stimulants including herbal supplements and coffee

Avoid all alcohol

Take supplements for short periods of time only

Take time out every day to rest and relax

Avoid too much external stimulation (parties, stress, etc)

Avoid cigarettes

Liver Qi Stagnation

Use spices that move the Qi throughout the body like peppermint, rosemary, spearmint, turmeric and thyme.

Be sure to chew your foods thoroughly before swallowing

Avoid overeating and hard to digest foods

Avoid foods containing preservatives or other chemicals

Always sit quietly while eating

Opt for smaller, more frequent meals

Avoid alcohol, caffeine and cigarettes

Get enough rest and exercise

Avoid emotional tension (anger, frustration, resentment).

Laugh more

Practice deep breathing exercises

Avoid hormonally treated meat and dairy products

Blood Stasis

Consume moderate amounts of soy and soy products

Eat only organic fruits and vegetables

Eat plenty of lemons, limes, onions, kelp, Irish moss and bladder wrack

Eat plenty of walnuts, chestnuts, chives, crabs, berries, broccoli, scallions, onions, beets, turnips, cauliflower and brussel sprouts.

Add grapes, lemons, tomatoes, cucumbers and celery to your diet

Avoid refined, hydrogenated oil

Use only unprocessed plant sources of essential fatty acids (nuts, seeds and dark green veggies)

Use oils rich in both linoleic and alpha-linoleic

Avoid sources of arachidonic acid which comes from animal meats, dairy products and peanuts.

Avoid animal products except fish

Avoid eating cold foods straight from the refrigerator or freezer

Do not put ice in your drinks.

Do not swim in cold water.

Do not use tampons.

Spleen Qi Deficiency

Consume mostly organic vegetables. To retain their nutritional value, be sure to sauté or lightly cook them.

Eat plenty of grains like brown rice, oats and sorghum.

Eat plenty of yams, pumpkin and pumpkin seeds, *unless* you suffer from PCOS.

Eat beef, chicken, goose, ham and mackerel.

Eat cherries, dates, figs and molasses.

Do not eat raw or cold foods.

Refrain from putting ice in your drinks or eating things straight from the refrigerator or freezer.

Avoid "cold" fruits and vegetables such as: mangoes, watermelon, pears, persimmons, cucumbers, lettuce, celery and spinach.

Avoid foods made from white flour.

Avoid sugar and all sugar substitutes

Avoid fruit juice.

Avoid dairy products (milk, cheese and ice cream)

Get plenty of rest and exercise

Avoid exercising during your period

Try meditation

Blood Deficiency

Eat plenty of these foods:

apricots, blueberries, raspberries and grapes

eggs

organic meats

turnips, watercress, and other dark leafy vegetables

hormone free liver and bone marrow

never smoke cigarettes

be sure to rest during your period

Phlegm-Damp accumulation

Eat lots of alfalfa, parsley, summer melons, radishes, carrots, celery, cranberries, cucumbers, lettuce and kelp.

Avoid greasy and fried foods

Avoid sugar, fruit juices and refined carbohydrates

Avoid all dairy products

Do not overindulge in soy products

Avoid wheat and wheat products

Avoid bananas, chocolate and nuts

Page 135

Heat deficiency

Eat plenty of foods that nourish the Blood and the Yin (beets and corn)

Avoid caffeine, artificial stimulants and cigarettes
Practice relaxation and deep breathing techniques at least once a day.
Perform Qi Gong Techniques regularly
Listen to quiet meditative tapes before bed.

Excess heat

Include cooling Yin-tonifying foods in your diet (plums, pears, tomatoes, and pomegranates)

Avoid all alcoholic drinks
Avoid spicy and greasy foods
Do not take hot baths
Avoid saunas and Jacuzzis

Step Three: Using Acupuncture, and TCM Herbs to Cleanse and Balance Your Energy for Conception

Acupuncture really does work when it comes to enhancing a woman's ability to conceive! Even Western medical practitioners are encouraging patients to give it a try.

According to researchers in the Fertility and Sterility journal published by the American Society for Reproductive Medicine (2002), a woman who undergoes acupuncture before IVF treatment is twice as likely to conceive as those who do not. The reason, according to acupuncture and acupressure experts is simple: it helps to relax the uterus; improve blood flow; and create a thicker endocrine lining, which are all needed to enhance conception.

What Acupuncture is All About

There's more to acupuncture than simply jabbing a patient with a bunch of needles. Used for thousands of years in Asia, acupuncture is used as a way to exchange the electrons within the bodies' meridians in order to help the body work more efficiently.

What Are the Meridians and How Do They Affect Fertility?

Meridians are lines of energy running through the body. They have a very unique affect on each of the body's separate systems – including the reproductive system.

How do your meridians affect your fertility? Before we can answer that question, we need to look at how the meridians themselves are formed in order to better understand their connection to the body's systems.

When an embryo is forming in a woman's womb, its cells are continually dividing. As these cells start to coalesce, they begin to create fold lines that separate different groups of cells and mark connections between those that are alike. Eventually these cell groups will form the body's internal organs. What's amazing is that these "folds" remain in our bodies long after we are born, connecting every group of cells together in a channels of "meridian energy connections." Even parts of the body which don't appear to be connected in any way really are because of these energy channels. This may explain why acupoints on the feet may or along the arms can actually affect your kidneys or even ovaries.

When electrical energy begins to encounter resistance, it can back-up, causing problems. Acupuncture is a good way to relieve this pressure and enhance proper energy flow once again.

When looking at the body, you will notice four main meridian groups connected to reproduction. They are called the Extraordinary Meridians:

The Penetrating Meridian

The Penetrating Meridian controls a woman's hormonal cycles, directing the Yin and Yang energies in the body.

The Conception Meridian (Yin)

The Conception Meridian regulates all of the bodies Yin meridians, which produces the estrogen her female system needs to work properly.

The Governing Meridian (Yang)

The governing Meridian oversees the production of Yang hormones such as progesterone and testosterone.

The Girdle Meridian

The Girdle Meridian is thought to encase the body horizontally around the midsection, like a girdle. It connects the penetrating and the conception meridians and helps to restrain vaginal leakage and miscarriage.

Although traditional fertility practitioners may encourage the use of acupuncture during fertility treatments, most do not completely understand how it works. Most attribute its positive effects to the release of chemicals that are stimulated by the nervous system during the procedure, while Eastern practitioners know full well that there is much more to the story of how the meridians affect a woman's fertility and use that knowledge to help break the cycle of infertility.

So, how does acupuncture work for aiding fertility? There are several theories:

Acupuncture needles stimulate the production of endorphins and help to rebalance the body's energies and aid in keeping all organs working at peak capacity.

The pressure exerted by the acupuncture needle actually creates a micro electric current in the body. This helps to release prostaglandins into the bloodstream and send messages to the hypothalamus, to regulate your hormones.

Note: **The stimulation of the pituitary gland** during acupuncture can benefit men also, helping to improve the concentration, volume and motility of their sperm.

It is important to remember when turning to acupuncture that different points have different effects, so the caregiver you choose to handle your treatment would be well qualified to treat your specific issues in order for it to work.

Sidebar: How Acupuncture Can Assist Pelvic Blood Flow – and why that's important

Most people understand the Importance of ovulation in order to get pregnant, but few understand the role that pelvic blood flow has in keeping the menstrual cycle on track and the ovaries healthy. To function at peak capacity, both the ovaries and the uterus must have adequate blood supply. Without it, they cannot form the protective cave necessary for an egg to be fertilized, implant and grow a baby. Therefore, poor blood flow can inhibit pregnancy.

Research has shown that acupuncture can reduce constriction of the uterine arteries, increase blood flow to the reproductive organs and thus increase a woman's chance of getting pregnant.

Note: To date, acupuncture is the only proven technique able to directly increase vascular response!"

How Acupressure Can Help

Both acupressure and acupuncture can help you get pregnant in two important ways:

By depressing the sympathetic nervous system.
By enhancing the effectiveness of other medical intervention methods.

The body is compiled of a system of reactions and feedback. Like a chain reaction, pressing on certain points or meridians can invigorate the blood and send messages to specific areas of the body that can enhance your fertility.

Although using acupuncture needles may offer the most help for many people, a lot are simply too squeamish for the procedure and opt for a less invasive acupressure treatment. Perfectly acceptable, acupressure employs the same basic techniques, only without the needles.

The other nice benefit of using acupressure is the fact that you can often stimulate the acupoints on your own body once you learn the proper technique and understand which points must be addressed in your own individual situation and treatment.

Although basic acupressure is most common, there are other therapy methods used by acupressurists that can also enhance your ability to get pregnant. They include:

Heat Therapy

Pressure points can be easily activated with warm compresses. Many Chinese practitioners use moxibustion (traditional Chinese medicine therapy using moxa, or mugwort herb. Suppliers usually age the mugwort and grind it up to a fluff; practitioners burn the fluff or process it further into a stick that resembles a (non-smokable) cigar. They can use it indirectly, with acupuncture needles, or sometimes burn it on a patient's skin.), to treat a cold uterus or other Yang deficiencies that may be found in the kidney or uterus. For those who have a lower abdomen that is cold to the touch, warming the uterus every day with a warm water bottle may help to stretch the capillaries and encourage blood flow.

Light Therapy

Light from the red spectrum of a pocket-sized light pen can be used to stimulate acupuncture points in the same way that needles do. Believe it or not, the light rays can actually penetrate the skin tissue and change the electrical potential (and the energy) of the cell. For best results touch the light to the skin's acupoint for five seconds.

Magnetic Therapy

Magnets are often used by practitioners to stimulate the body electromagnetically, and increase circulation. For best results, tape the magnets right to the skin above the acupoint you are treating.

Since it can be quite complicated to figure out which acupoints to address (and how) for the average layperson, it is usually best to visit with a licensed acupressurists in order to set up a treatment plan and learn what acupressure points and moves will be best for you.

However, it is possible to figure out which points to focus on and treat yourself. In order to figure out which points to apply proper pressure, you must remember the basics of the meridians points and organs, as well as your diagnosis. Remember, there are 12 major meridians running through your body, and each meridian (or channel) runs to and through a specific organ system. These 12 are usually described in pairs since they link energy systems to organs:

Lung (Yin) is paired with the large intestine (Yang)

Heart (Yin) is paired with the small intestine (Yang)

Pericardium (Yin) is paired with the Triple Warmer (Yang)

Spleen (Yin) is paired with the stomach (Yang)

Kidney (Yin) is paired with the bladder (Yang)

Liver (Yin) is paired with the gallbladder (Yang)

Once you know your diagnosis, you can manipulate the points within that category. But remember, it's important to draw the body's attention and energies to the reproductive organs, regardless of the overall diagnosis when using this type of treatment.

Main Acupuncture
Points to Focus On

Ear Triangular Fossa

Found in the upper, inner part of the ear, outing pressure on the Triangular Fossa can help to stimulate the Uterus and fallopian tubes. It's best to massage this area whenever you feel stressed.

Ear Intertragic Notch

The ear intertragic notch (located just above the earlobe in the crevice between the two cartilaginous areas in the lowest point inside of the ear), the Interlock Notch is used to treat the endocrine system and ovaries. For best results, massage this area once every day or two.

Epang II: Scalp Reproductive Points

Found in the scalp just above the forehead, on the inside upper corner of the hairline above the outside of the eyebrow, this important scalp point connects to the kidney energies, which help to regulate menstruation and other reproductive and pelvic functions.

Zigong (Palace of the Child)

Located about four inches below the navel and three inches lateral to the midline (near the ovaries), stimulating the Zigong can alleviate many common menstrual problems including cervical stenosis.

Ren 3 (Central Pole of the Conception Meridian)

Considered the North Star of the Conception meridian, Ren 3 regulates menstruation, kidney function, the bladder and staves off dampness and stagnation of the pelvis. It can also help to alleviate endometriosis. Ren 3 is found on the midline, about four inches below the navel. For best results massage using deep, circular motions before ovulation (only). Some people also use heat, light and magnet therapy to treat this point.

Ren 4 (Origin of the Source of the Conception Meridian)

Located at the site of the uterus (about four inches below the navel), Ren 4 is known to fortify the Qi, and assist in conception. For best results, massage using deep circular motions between your period and ovulation.

St 30 (Rushing Qi)

This point (located on the lower abdomen about five inches below the navel just above the pubic region), is known to penetrate the ovaries, fallopian tubes and uterus. For best results use circular massage methods with light and heat stimulation.

KI 16 (Vitals Shu)

A transmitter of the immune system, Ki 16 stimulation can get rid of any energy blocks in the abdomen which may be interfering with conception. For best results, massage in a circular motion while applying heat, light or magnets.

For a breakdown of the points needed to be stimulated for individual fertility problems see the following descriptions and illustrations:

Points to Enhance the Kidney (Yin)

The following points can be used to tonify the kidney Yin:

KI 3 (Great Ravine) —This point clears heat and strengthens the kidney energies

KI 6 (Shining Sea) – used to cool the blood and treat infertility heat issues

Lu 7 (Broken Sequence) -- this point regulates the conception meridian and controls water balance within the body

Sp 6 (Joining of the three Yin) – The culminating point for all of the Yin channels (kidney, spleen and liver), this leg point helps to regulate menstruation

UB 23 (Back Point of the Kidney) – The main point of the kidney's energies, helps to tonify both the Yin and the Yang energies.

Additional important points to focus on:

KI-2 Rangu

Points to Enhance the Kidney (Yang)

The following points are used to tonify the Kidney's Yang and relieve a cold uterus:

KI 7 – This point is used to treat scarred fallopian tubes

ST 36 – Primarily a stomach and spleen point, it is used to treat gastrointestinal disorders

Du 4 (Life Gate) – Said to reside between the two kidneys, this point is known to affect the womb and strengthen the Qi and the Kidney Yang in order to resolve cold issues and impotence.

Ren 6 – Used to help overcome fatigue and enhances Qi

SI 3 – Helps to open the governing meridian

Additional important points to focus on:

KI-3 Taixi

BL-23 Shenshu

Ren-3 Zhongji

BL-32 Ciliao and the other Baliao

Ren-4 Guanyuan

Points to Treat Elevated Hormone Levels

Yintang- helps with headaches and anxiety but also lowers excess prolactin levels.

LI 4 -used to lower excess prolactin levels.

Lv 2 -used to lower excess prolactin levels.

Lv 3 -used to lower excess prolactin levels.

UB 2, UB 62 and Si 3 can be used to level pituitary hormones.

Points to Treat Stagnate Liver Qi

Lv 14 – this point treats menstrual chills, breasts pain and sensitivity and enhances liver Qi.

Lv 2 – this point is used to remove excess hormones and heat from the heart.

Lv 3 – this point helps to regulate menstruation, treat low sperm and stagnant liver Qi.

Additional important points to focus on:

PC-7 Daling
HE-5 Tongli
HE-7 Shenmen
PC-6 Neiguan

Points to Nourish the Blood

Lv 8 – helps to treat dampness in reproductive system and regulate your period.

Sp 6 - (Joining of the three Yin) – The culminating point for all of the Yin channels (kidney, spleen and liver), this leg point helps to regulate menstruation

St 36 – Primarily a stomach and spleen point, it is used to treat gastrointestinal disorders.

Points to Treat Stagnate Blood

Sp 10 (Sea of Blood) – helps to cool the blood and treat clotting, uterine fibroids and dark menstrual flow.

UB 17 – used to cool hot blood, resolve blood stasis and treat abnormal bleeding

Sp 6 - (Joining of the three Yin) – The culminating point for all of the Yin channels (kidney, spleen and liver), this leg point helps to regulate menstruation.

Additional important points to focus on:

Ren-4

Ren-2

ST-29

ST-36

SP-6

LIV-5

Points to Treat Phlegm-Damp Accumulation

St 40 – Used to treat polycystic ovaries, obstructions of the fallopian tubes and accumulated dampness in the pelvis.

Ren 3 – regulates menstruation, kidney function, the bladder and staves off dampness and stagnation of the pelvis.

Ren 12 – treats dampness caused by weakened spleen.

Additional important points to focus on:

Ren-6 Qihai
GB-26 Daimai
SP-5 Shangqui
BL-28 Pangguangshu

Points to Treat Bleeding from the Uterus

KI 8 – used to treat uterine bleeding due to blood stasis.

Sp 8 –this point promotes circulation of blood at ovulation and regular periods.

Du 20 – helps to alleviate a spleen deficiency

Points to Increase Blood Flow to the Pelvic Organs

Sp 6 -(Joining of the three Yin) – The culminating point for all of the Yin channels (kidney, spleen and liver), this leg point helps to regulate menstruation

UB 23- The main point of the kidney's energies, helps to tonify both the Yin and the Yang energies.

UB 52— used to treat low libido, impotence and menstrual problems.

UB 31-regulates menstruation and enhancing blood flow to pelvic organs

UB 31-regulates menstruation and enhancing blood flow to pelvic organs

UB 33- regulates menstruation and enhancing blood flow to pelvic organs

UB 34- regulates menstruation and enhancing blood flow to pelvic organs

Points to Treat the Spleen

Ren 6 – Used to help overcome fatigue and enhances Qi

Sp 6 -(Joining of the three Yin) – The culminating point for all of the Yin channels
(kidney, spleen and liver), this leg point helps to regulate menstruation

ST 36 – Primarily a stomach and spleen point, it is used to treat gastrointestinal
disorders

Points to Treat the Heart

UB 44—reduces excess heat from the heart, enhances kidney function and regulates Qi.

Ub 15 regulates the heart's Qi, calms anxiety, helps blood stasis and reduces excess heat from the heart.

Ren 14- Treats obsessions, anxiety and fears.

Additional important points to focus on:

HE-5 Tongli
PC-7 Daling
HE-7 Shenmen
PC-6 Neiguan

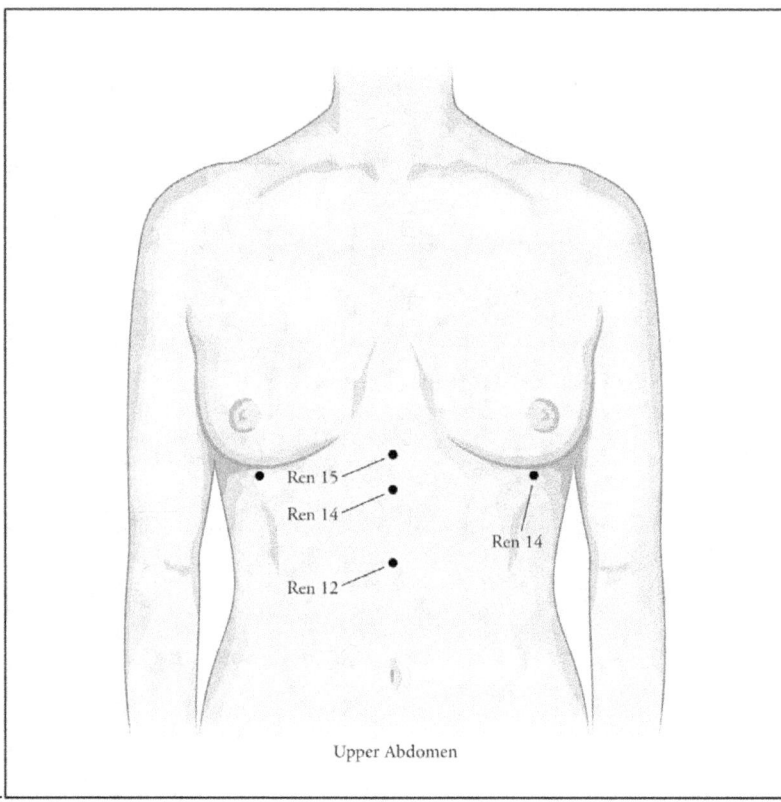

Upper Abdomen

Figure 2: Upper Abdomen Acupoints

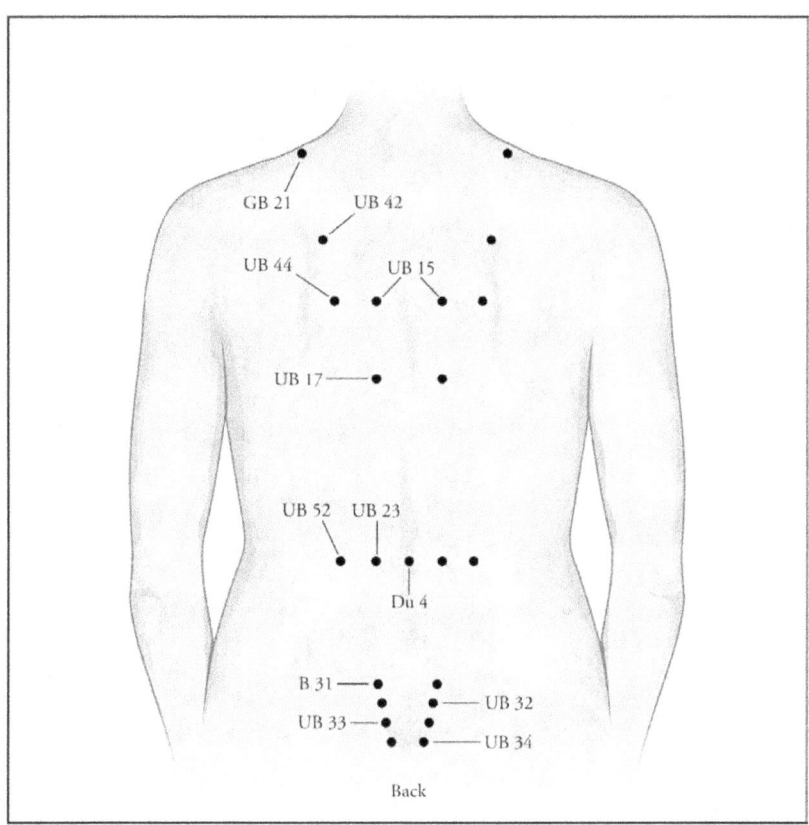

Figure 3: Back Acupoints

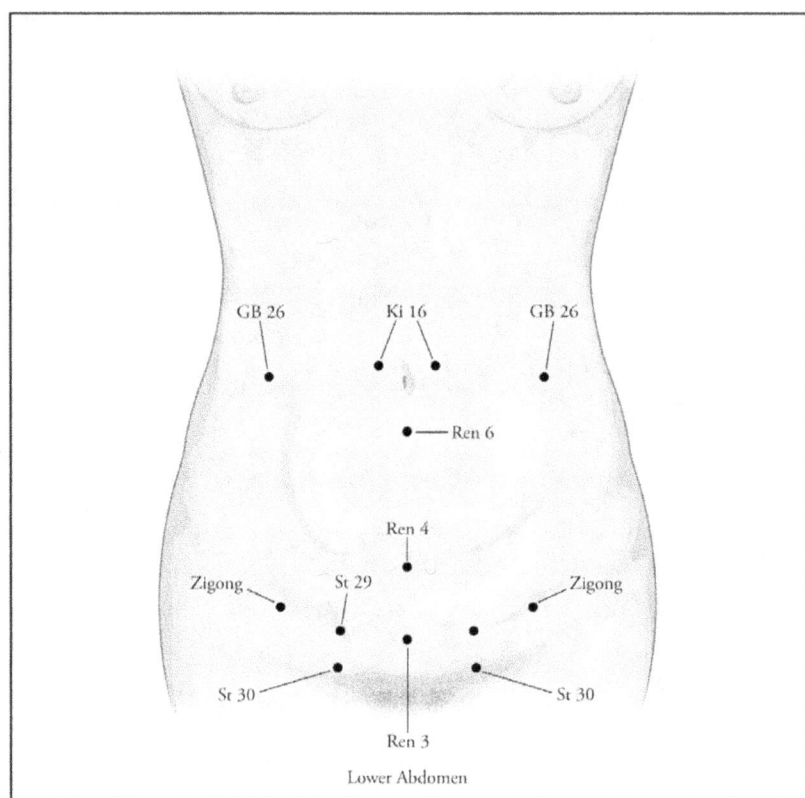

Lower Abdomen

Figure 4: Lower Abdomen Acupoints

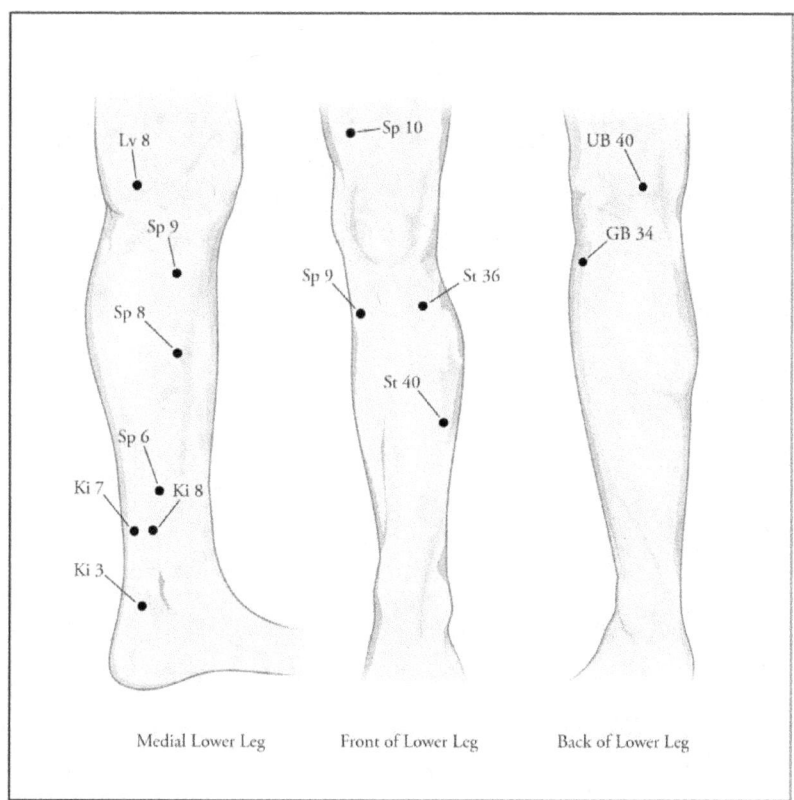

Figure 5: Leg Acupoints

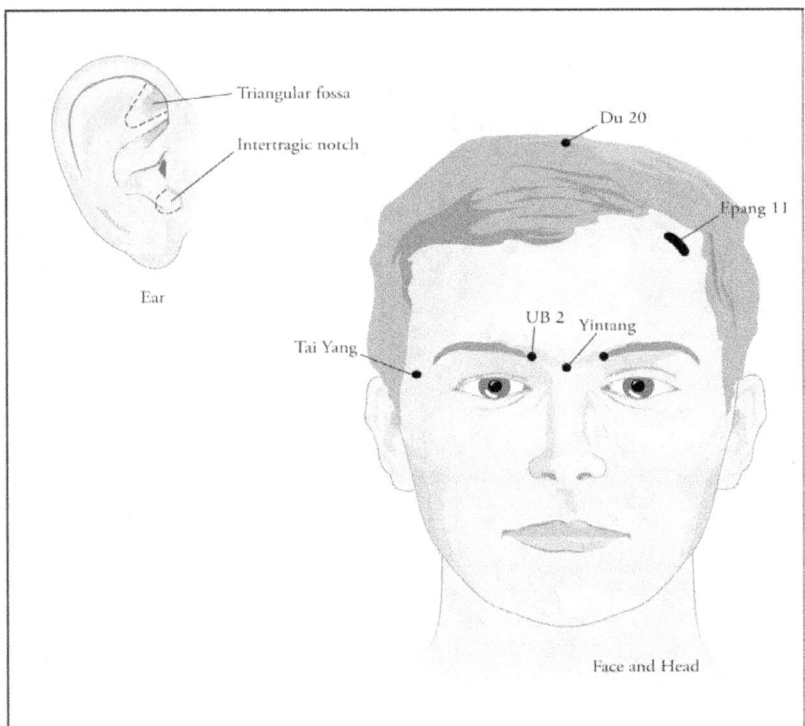

Figure 6: Face and Head Acupoints

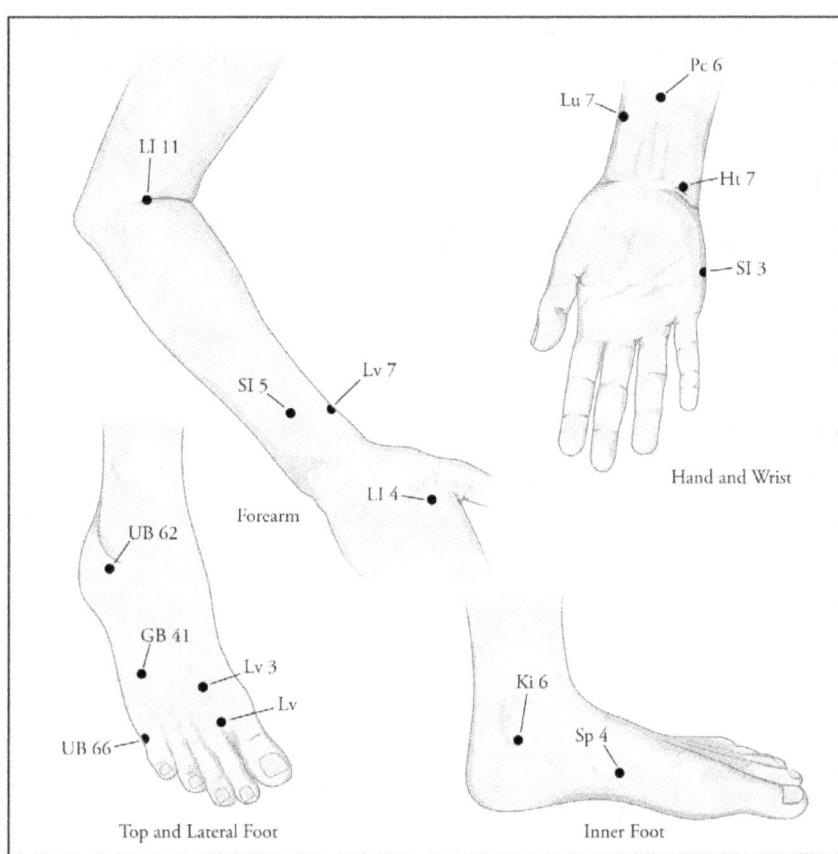

Figure 7: Hand and Foot Acupoints

Page 163

Although some people prefer to use stones or other implements to massage the skin, simple massage using the fingertips, thumb and/or a small rubber mallet works best for most.

When using acupressure be sure to apply enough pressure with the tip of your finger to create a slight aching or full sensation at the desired pressure point area.

Abdominal points should be massaged in deep, clockwise, circular motions for a few minutes every other day before ovulation for best results.

Energy Balancing Herbs

While acupuncture and acupressure are used to balance the body's energies externally, herbs are used to balance the body's internal energies.   They can be used to restore hormone imbalances, and encourage ovulation.

One of the main differences between herbal therapy and traditional drug therapy is the fact that pharmaceuticals are created to treat symptoms; while herbs are used to treat the causes of those symptoms.

The second difference that should be addressed – especially for women trying to get pregnant – is the side effects of using pharmaceuticals instead of herbs. Pharmaceutical medications are always accompanied with a list of possible side effects. Some show up right away, while others may not present themselves for weeks months or even years. Herbs, on the other hand, are completely natural, and used not to change the molecular formula of the body (as drugs do), but to coax the body into producing its own healing substances and energies.

Of course, not every herb can _- or should – be used by every woman, even if they seem to suffer from the same ailment.   We've already discussed how every couple's fertility problems stem from their own unique organ deficiencies. There are specific herbs designed to deal with each specific problem, whether it be Yin, Yang, blood or some other Qi energy issue.   For instance, some herbs stimulate, while other herbs calm. So be absolutely certain that any herbs you are taking have been approved by your herbalist; Traditional Chinese Medicine physicians and/or your regular OBGYN.

When using herbs, remember this important tip: they should be used in their raw form as much as possible. Although pills and powder form are available – and can be useful – most experts agree that the raw form of herbs is always more effective.

Which herbs you are prescribed will depend a great deal on what stage of your menstrual cycle needs a boost. However, here is a rundown of the most common herbs given to women who are trying to get pregnant:

Liquid Chlorophyll

Chlorophyll is the natural substance that makes the green color of plants and leaves. Chlorophyll is rich in magnesium, copper, iron, protein, vitamin A, potassium, sodium, calcium, vitamin E, lithium, phosphorus, zinc and a number of other essential nutrients. It is often said that chlorophyll in plants works like blood does in the human body. The primary source of dietary chlorophyll is green leafy vegetables. However, most of the chlorophyll in plants is lost during the cooking process, ultimately leaving a very little amount that is not enough to provide any significant health benefits. Therefore it is better to obtain chlorophyll from dietary supplements.

It enhances the work of hemoglobin in our blood and helps to replenish the amount of red blood cells in our body. By doing so, it aids in the growth and maintenance of tissues, and helps to heal wounds more effectively. It is an antiseptic, and inhibits the growth of bacteria in the body.

Chlorophyll is known to neutralize the polluted air that is breathed in the body every day.

Another benefit of chlorophyll is in chelating toxic metals and heavy minerals in the body, such as mercury and calcium. It is also used to cleanse the liver, regulate menstruation and build up the blood.

Astragalus

Astragalus is the root of A. membranaceus, members of the pea family native to northeast China. In China, the root is called huang-qi.

It has been used to invigorate vital energy (qi) and in prescriptions for shortness of breath, general weakness, and lack of appetite; also as a diuretic, and for the treatment of colds, flu, stomach ulcers, and diabetes. It is also known for stimulating the immune system and increasing sperm motility up to 150%.

Wild Yams

Wild yams, or Dioscorea villosa, have a long history as a natural pain reliever.

The wild yamsn plant is also known as colic root or rheumatism root and has a long history of both medicinal and culinary use. It is used to enhance fertility due to containing steroid-like compounds which are easily converted into sex hormones in the body, triggering the release of FSH which stimulates the ovaries to release an egg. High yam consumption appears to stimulate release of more than one egg each month (causing twins). Can be purchased and used in cream form.

Pumpkin Seeds

In traditional Chinese medicine, pumpkin seeds have sweet and neutral properties and are associated with the Large Intestine and Stomach meridians. They are often used to alleviate pain and expel parasites.

The recommended daily dosage for pumpkin seed, unless otherwise prescribed, is 10 grams of whole and coarsely ground seed for internal uses. Taken with fluids, in the morning and evening. It is recommended that the testa, the seed's outer covering, be removed before consumption.

Rich in zinc, it is a nutrient vital to healthy functioning of the male reproductive system.

Agnus Castus (Chaste tree berry)

The herb of choice for promoting hormone balance within the body and regulating your period; increasing the ratio of progesterone to estrogen and balancing excess estrogen.

Studies have shown that extracts of Agnus castus can stimulate the release of Leutenizing Hormone (LH) and inhibit the release of Follicle Stimulating Hormone (FSH). This suggests that the volatile oil has a progesterone-like effect. Its benefits stem from its actions upon the pituitary gland specifically on the production of luteinizing hormone. This increases progesterone production and helps regulate a woman's cycle. The ability to decrease excessive prolactin levels may benefit infertile women.

Blessed Thistle

Cnicus benedictus (St. Benedict's thistle or spotted thistle and it is not the same as milk thistle). It has sometimes been used as a galactogogue to promote lactation. The crude drug contains about 0.2% cnicin. It is recommended for use by public health nurses in Ontario, Canada, as well as by the Canadian Breastfeeding Foundation to increase lactation in nursing mothers. It is also a hormone balancer used for general female problems.

Red Raspberry Leaves

The red raspberry leaf (Rubus idaeus) is produced by the raspberry plant and has traditional medical uses due to its rich content in vitamins, minerals, and tannins.

It is recommended to pregnant women, especially as an aid in delivery. The red raspberry leaf also contains many essential minerals such as phosphorus, potassium, and an easily assimilated form of calcium. It also contains fragrine, an alkaloid which help tone the muscles of the pelvic region including the uterus.

Page 169

False Unicorn Root

False Unicorn Root is a summer-flowering plant that was first used by Native North Americans to prevent miscarriage, expel worms and to treat liver and kidney ailments, and had become an important domestic remedy for depression, infertility and the "derangements of women" .False Unicorn Root appears to have its greatest value in female disorders of the reproductive organs. The herb is said to stimulate ovarian hormones and may be helpful in cases of early menopause after hysterectomy or to restart the system after years of contraception (giving some credence to its historic use as a fertility aid).   In addition, it is also said to relieve vaginal dryness, hot flashes, night sweats, mood swings and depression (also echoing its past use in herbal medicine), as well as other symptoms related to menopause.

False Unicorn Root is said to relieve menstrual difficulties, fibroids, infertility, vaginal discharge, prolapsed uterus, endometriosis, pelvic inflammatory disease and threatened miscarriage.

Referred to as "the" herb for infertility. Take 5-15 drops of the tincture per day during the pre-conception period to strengthen the uterine muscle.

Evening Primrose Oil

Evening Primrose Oil has been called the most sensational preventive discovery since vitamin C. It contains the pain relieving compound phenylalanine and is increasingly being used to treat chronic headaches. It is currently being studied all over the world as a treatment for aging problems, alcoholism, acne, heart disease, hyperactivity in children, multiple sclerosis, weight control, obesity, PMS and schizophrenia.

Evening Primrose Oil contains a high concentration of a fatty acid called GLA and it is this fatty acid that is largely responsible for the remarkable healing properties of the plant. These fatty acids also help to regulate hormones and improve nerve function aiding problems ranging from PMS to migraine headaches. The hormone balancing effect contributes to healthy breast tissue.

Specifically, evening primrose oil may help to:

Relieve endometriosis and fibrocystic breasts: By interfering with the production of inflammatory prostaglandins released during menstruation. The oil's essential fatty acids can minimise breast inflammation and promote the absorption of iodine, a mineral that can be present in abnormally low levels in women with this condition.

Helps to increase fertile quality cervical fluid. Use from menstruation to ovulation, switching to Flax Seed Oil after ovulation.

Black Cohosh

Black cohosh (known as both Actaea racemosa and Cimicifuga racemosa), is used for hot flashes and other menopausal symptoms. It is recommended for menopausal symptoms, being hormone balancing herb that suppresses the secretion of luteinizing hormone and has estrogenic effects.

Damiana

Damiana is used as a general tonic for the nervous, hormonal, and reproductive systems. It has an ancient reputation as an aphrodisiac. Damiana has long been claimed to have a stimulating effect on libido, and its use as an aphrodisiac has continued into modern times. It has also been shown that damiana may function as an aromatase, which has been suggested as a possible method of action for its reputed effects. Used to enhance fertility and sexual desire in both sexes.

Kelp

Kelp refers to several species of large, brown algae. The large amounts of iodine found in Kelp are important in the treatment of an under-active thyroid. Consequently, Kelp may contribute to weight loss if the weight gain is directly related to thyroid disorders. Kelp helps improve digestion, stimulate kidney function, increase circulation, and purify the blood. Kelp has also been known to treat inflamed joints and tissues caused by arthritis & rheumatism. Furthermore, Kelp enhances the immune system and eliminates the negative effects that stress may have on the body. Kelp has natural organic antibiotics and is also used to prevent miscarriage.

Ho Shou Wu

This remarkable herb possesses properties similar to ginseng. It increases strength in the liver and kidneys as well as the bones and muscles. It is known to calm the nervous system and clear the eyes.

Its strength comes from the actions of cleansing the liver and kidneys. It's ability to increase energy, preserve youth and restore impaired sexual functioning has made it a favorite ingredient in Chinese patent medicine.

More current research has found it to be effective in reducing cholesterol levels, doubtless due to the lecithin found in the root.

Also used for lower back pain, insomnia, premature hair loss and graying, diabetes and hypo-glycemia. It also strengthens muscles, tendons, ligaments and bones.

Studies demonstrate its beneficial effects on fertility and ovulation.

Clover (Dong Quai Root)

Helps to normalize the menstrual cycles. Use between ovulation and menstruation only.

Dong Quai is also known as Chinese Angelica and is primarily known for it's uses in treating women's problems including lack of sexual desire, the symptoms of menopause, cramps and PMS. It aids in increasing the effects of hormones in both men and women and is widely used as an aphrodisiac. Dong Quai is particularly useful in helping to end hot flashes and menstrual cramps. It is also used as a liver tonic and in treating sciatica and shingles. It is traditionally characterized as a warm atmospheric energy that promotes blood circulation.

Using Chinese Herbs to Treat Infertility

For centuries Chinese practitioners have been developing the proper use of herbs in helping women achieve their maximum fertility. This is done mainly by utilizing the properties in specific herbs to harmonize the endocrine system.

Of course different herbs work on different organ systems, so it is important to understand how each herb works independently, as well as in conjunction with others you may be taking.

One of the main differences between Chinese herbal treatments, and traditional medicines is the fact that a Chinese practitioner does not treat individual symptoms, but rather the underlying reason for the imbalance which is causing the symptom. The treatment is designed to fit the pattern, not the disease. Here are a few guidelines to follow when using Chinese herbal therapy:
Choose herbs that are based on your symptoms, BBT chart results and diagnosis pattern.

For instance, the following treatments may be considered for these ailments:

Kidney Yin Deficiency -- Kidney Yin Tonics

Kidney Yin and Yang Deficiency – Kidney Essence Tonics

Kidney Yang Deficiency – Kidney Yang Tonics

Spleen Qi Deficiency – Spleen Qi Supplements

Blood Deficiency – Blood Builders

Heart Deficiency – Heart Supplements

Blood Stasis – Blood Movers

Liver Qi Stagnation – Liver Qi Movers

Excess heat – Heat Clearers

Phlegm-Damp accumulation– Damp Drainers

Damp Heat – Damp Heat Resolves

General Instructions:

Treat Multiple Patterns Concurrently.
Adjust formulas when side effects occur to eliminate creating new diagnosis patterns by inducing new deficiencies.
Be consistent, accurate and patient with treatment.
Be sure to tell your doctor about every treatment you use (including herbal therapy).

Chinese herbs are used depending on your underlying diagnostic category during different phases of your menstrual cycle. Here is a quick rundown of what treatments should be administered when:

Phase I (the follicular stage) – It is best to nourish the blood and Yin during this time of the month
Phase II (ovulation) – Use herbs to move the Qi and blood and keep levels adequate
Phase III (premenstrual phase) – use herbs to keep liver Qi from stagnating
Phase V (menstruation) – Take nothing during this time. Menstruation is considered a zero hormonal period, and should be used as a time of rest for you and your body.

The following herbs can be used to treat the conditions specified. But remember, as with any medicine, it is important to take cues from your body and watch for side effects or adverse reactions. Herbal therapy isn't instantaneous and you can't expect results right away. But, if you are patient (and continue to listen to what your body is telling you), you can expect some improvement soon.

Kidney Yin Tonics

Yin-tonifying herbs are used from the end of the blood phase to ovulation and help the body produce the right amount of hormones.

Tian Men Dong (asparagus root) –used to nourish the Yin of the Kidney and Lung.   Dosage: 12 grams

Mai Men Dong (Ophiopogon root) – used to moisten the lungs and augment stomach Yin. Dosage: 12 grams

Han Lian Cao (Eclipta) – used to cool the blood and nourish the liver and kidney Yin.   Dosage: 12 grams

Nu Zhen Zi (Ligustrum, privet fruit) – used to nourish the Liver and Kidney Yin. Dosage: 10 grams

He Shou Wu (Solomon's Seel Root) – used to tonify the kidneys and liver and blood essence. Dosage: 15 grams

Sang Ji Sheng (Loranthus, mulberry, mistletoe) – helps to tonify the kidneys and liver; nourishes the blood; relaxes the uterus during pregnancy; and strengthens the bones. Helps to prevent miscarriage and lower blood pressure. Dosage: 15 grams.

Other herbs to focus on:

Long Yan Rou 10 g Arillus Euphoriae Longanae

Fu Shen 6 g Sclerotium Poriae Cocos Pararadicis

Shu Di 12 g Radix Rehmanniae Glutinosae Conquitae

Sheng Di 12 g Radix Rehmanniae Glutinosae

Shan Zhu Yu 10 g Fructus Corni Officinalis

Shan Yao 10 g Dioscorea Oppositae

Suan Zao Ren 15 g Semen Ziziphi Spinosae

Bai Zi Ren 10 g Semen Biotae Orientalis

Dang Gui 10 g Radix Angelicae Sinensis

Ze Xie 5 g Rhizoma Alismatis

Mu Dan Pi 6 g Cortex Moutan Radicis

Chinese Patent Formulas to Tonify Kidney Yin

Liu Wei Huang Wan.
Zhi Bai Di Huang Wan

Kidney Essence Tonics

These tonics are used to stabilize kidney essence and raise the reproductive Qi:

Helonias (false unicorn root) – helps to retain the essence of both the Yin and the Yang and nourish the reproductive Qi in order to treat low progesterone levels, low fertility, miscarriage and excessive vaginal discharge. Dosage: 7 grams. (Note: do not take if you experience scant cervical mucus).

Fu Pen Zi (Chinese raspberry) – used to stabilize the kidneys, preserve the essence and assist the Yang energies. Dosage: 7 grams.

Shan Zhu Yu (Cornus, Asian Corenlian cherry fruit) -- helps to stabilize the kidneys and extend reproductive function and tonify the Yang to treat low sperm motility and excessive menstruation. Dosage: 7 grams.

Kidney Yang Tonics

Since Kidney Yang energies are warm energies, using these tonics will add heat to the system, so care should be taken if you experience other heat symptoms since this treatment can make your symptoms worse. These tonics can be used successfully to increase thyroid hormone and progesterone production:

Man Jing Zi (chaste tree berry, Vitex fruit) – used to help the body produce more LH hormone, while prohibiting the release of FSH. Can also be used to inhibit the production of prolactin, which can stop ovulation from occurring. Dosage: 300 milligrams per day in tablet form.

Damiana Mexican Wild Yam – used to tonify the reproductive Qi and the Yang. Dosage: 6 grams infusion; 2 milliliters tincture.

Saw Palmetto – used to enhance the pituitary function and nourish the reproductive Qi to treat impotence, amenorrhea, long menstrual cycles and a lack of sexual desire. Dosage: 6 grams dry; 2 milliliters in tincture form.

Ba Ji Tian (Morinda Root) – used to strengthen and warm the reproductive system. Dosage: 12 grams

Yin Yang Huo (Epimedium goatweed) – used to tonify deficient kidney Yang in order to treat low libido and premature ejaculation. Dosage: 9 grams.

Xian Mao (Immortal grass, goldenye grass) – warms the kidney Yang to treat a cold uterus and impotence. Note: for short term use only. Dosage: 6 grams.

Du Zhong (Encomia bark) – used to promote circulation and treat cold Yang deficiency to prevent miscarriage. Dosage: 12 grams.

Xu Duan (Japanese teasel root) – used to tonify the kidneys and liver to treat cramping, bleeding and prevent miscarriage. Dosage: 15 grams.

Bou Cong Rong (Broomrape stem) -- used to tonify the Kidney Yang to treat a cold uterus and impotence. Dosage: 15 grams.

Other herbs to focus on:

Tu Si Zi 10 g Semen Cuscatae

Rou Cong Rong 5 g Herba Cistanches

Patent Chinese Herbal Formulas Used to Tonify the

Kidney yang:

Eight Ingredient Pill with Rehmannia
Kidney Qi Pill
Two Immortals Decoction

Spleen Qi Supplements

A weak Qi will cause havoc in all systems, and a weakened Spleen Qi is no exception. These supplements can be very harsh to a compromised digestive track, so start treatment slowly to eliminate nausea and bloating. They are generally used to treat blood disorders:

Ren Shen (ginseng root) -- helps to boost immunity by strengthening the Qi to treat low sperm count, low testosterone and other immune disorders. Dosage: 6 grams. Note: Korean Ginseng is stronger than Chinese Ginseng.

American Ginseng – used to treat concurrent Qi and Yang deficiency. Dosage: 6 grams.

Siberian Ginseng – protects and regulates the immune system and is great for treating low energy and an inability to deal with stress. Dosage: 3 grams.

Dang Shen (Codonopis Root) – used to augment Qi. Dosage: 15 grams.

Huang Qi (Astragals Root) – used to tonify the spleen Qi and raise Yang Qi. Dosage: 15 grams.

Shan Yao (Chinese yam) – helps to increase spleen energy and preserve kidney function. Dosage: 15 grams.

Bai Zhu (Atracylodes) – used to enhance spleen Qi and dry dampness. Dosage: 6 grams.

Patent Chinese Herbal Formulas Used to Treat

Spleen Qi Deficiencies

Augment Qi Decoction
Four gentlemen Decoction

Heart Nourishing Herbs

Mu Li- helps with insomnia, restlessness. Calms the spirit.
Dosage: 20 grams.

Zao Ren- Lowers body temperature, calms the spirit and nourishes the heart
Dosage: 20 grams.

Patent Chinese Herbal Formulas Used

to Tonify and Calm the Heart

Tian Wang Bu Xin Dang
Sour Jujube Decoction

Phlegm-Damp Accumulation Herbs

Hai Zao – helps to reduce dampness and excess heat. Helps with high cholesterol and clotting. Dosage: 10 grams.

Fu Ling- helps to relax the nervous system, enhance the spleen and remove excess dampness. Dosage: 12 grams.

Other Dampness Clearing Herbs to Focus On

Ba Ji Tian 5 g Radix Morindae Officinalis

Yi Yi Ren 15 g Semen Coicis Lachryma-jobi

Sha Ren 6 g Fructus seu Semen Amomi

Tu Si Zi 10 g Semen Cuscatae

Xu Duan 5 g Radix Dipsaci

Nu Zhen Zi 10 g Fructus Ligustri Lucidi

Han Lian Cao 10 g Herba Ecliptae Prostratae

Ji Xue Teng 12 g Radix et Caulis Jixueteng

Patent Chinese Herbal Formulas Used

to Remove Damp Accumulation

Two Cured Decodation

Blood Builders

Taking these blood building herbs can help improve uterine lining and ovarian response, and thus increase fertility.

Dang Gui, Dong Quai (Angelica) – helps to nourish and invigorate the blood to treat menstrual issues. Dosage: 9 grams. Note: Do not take if you are already taking blood thinners.

Shu Juang (Cooked Rehmania, Chinese foxglove root) -- used to tonify the blood and essence and boorish the kidney Yin to treat heat conditions. Dosage: 15 grams.

Nettles – used to restore deficient liver blood and Yin by detoxifying the blood. Dosage: 15 grams pr 5-milliliter tincture.

Qi/BL – Herbs to Supplement Qi and Blood

The Qi travels through the blood, making it important to nourish both to ensure proper Yin and Yang balance. Try these herbs for nourishing both the Qi and the blood:

Avena Sativa, Oat Berry and Straw – used to nourish the endocrine and nervous systems and tonify the blood, Qi and essence in order to treat impotence, PMS and endocrine issues. Dosage: 20 grams.

Liver Qi Movers

The following herbs are used to remove energy blockages throughout the body and eliminate any stagnation:

Chai Hu- helps to enhance liver Qi , lifts the spirit and helps with gastro-intestinal disorders. Dosage: 7 grams.

Sheng Ma (black cohosh) – helps to raise the Yang Qi and vent heat. Dosage: 6 grams.

Chen PI (dried tangerine peel) – used to regulate Spleen Qi and prevent all types of stagnation. Dosage: 6 grams.

Xiang Fu (Cyprus) – used to spread and regulate the Liver Qi. Dosage: 9 grams.

Milk Thistle Seed – used to purify the blood and stimulate the uterus and can help the liver metabolize excess hormones and environmental toxins. Dosage: 600 milligrams per day.

Other Liver Qi Herbs to Focus On

Mu Li 15 g Concha Ostreae

Huang Lian 3 g Rhizoma Coptidis

Zhi Zi 5 g Fructus Gardeniae Jasminoidis

He Huan Pi 12 g Cortex Albizziae Julibrissin

Bai Zi Ren 10 g Semen Biotae Orientalis

Lian Zi Xin 1.5–3 g Plumula Nelumbinis Nuciferae

Suan Zao Ren 12 g Semen Ziziphi Spinosae

Chuan Lian Zi 5 g Fructus Meliae Toosendan

Patent Chinese Herbal Formulas to Help Move the

Liver Qi

Frigid Extremities Powder
Rambling Powder

Blood Movers

When a woman suffers from endometriosis or fibroids, these blood movers can be used to cleanse the uterus. Note: these herbs are blood thinners and should be utilized with care. See your doctor and TCM specialist for more details on their proper use.

Yi MU Cao (Leonurus, Chinese Motherwort) -- helps to regulate menses by invigorating the blood of the heart, liver and bladder. Dosage: 30 grams.

Tao Ren (peach kernel) – helps to break up blood stasis that may be preventing egg implantation. Note: never use after ovulation or if you are pregnant. Dosage: 6 grams.

Hong Hua (safflower) – used to unblock menstruation and treat amenorrhea. Dosage: 6 grams.

Blue Cohosh Root – used to raise estrogen levels and warm the uterus. Dosage: 6 grams; 2 milliliters tincture

Patent Chinese Herbal Formulas Used to Move the

Blood

Four Substances Decoction with Safflower and Peach Pit
Warm the Menses Decoction
Cinnamon Twig and Poria Decoction

Heat Clearing Herbs

Many infertility issues including short cycles and repeat miscarriage are caused by heat issues and can be resolved with these herbs:

Di Gu Pl (Chinese Wolfberry root bark) – used to clear heat from a Yin deficiency. Dosage: 10 grams

Chi Shao (red peony) – used to clear heat and cool and invigorate the blood to treat blood stasis and endometriosis. Dosage: 6 grams.

Mu Dan Pl (peony root bark) – used to clear heat and cool the blood to treat a variety of reproductive problems. Dosage: 9 grams.

Herbs to Drain Damp Heat

Huang Qin (skullcap root) – used to clear dampness from the upper body. Dosage: 6 grams

Hunag Lian (Coptis) – used to clear heat from the middle section of the body. Dosage: 4.5 grams.

Hunang Bai (Amur cork bark) – used to drain damp heat from the lower body and treat cervical inflammation. Dosage: 7 grams.

Calming Herbs to Prevent Miscarriage

These herbs offer a calming effect to a fetus, which can help to stave off miscarriage:

Atracylodes – used to tonify the Qi.

Gelatin -- used to tonify the blood and stop bleeding.

Dispacus – used to tonify the liver and kidneys.

Scutellaria – used to clear damp heat from the body.

Encomia – used to tonify kidney yang.

Perilla Fruit – used to warm and harmonize the spleen to treat cold conditions.

Artemisia – helps to warm the womb and stop bleeding. Can also treat a cold uterus and build up the uterine lining.

Page 192

Herbs to Help the Fallopian Tubes

Herbal medicine alone can't fix a blocked fallopian tube, however, if they are only sluggish or partially blocked these herbs may help to clear them in addition to other TCM treatments:

Playcodon (Jte Geng) – helps to get the egg through the fallopian tubes and into the uterus.

Tribulus -- used to reduce swelling and help heal damaged tissue.

Astragals – used to help heal tissue.

Herbs Used to Stop Bleeding

Bulrush (cattail pollen) – used to invigorate static blood.

Agrimonia – used to treat bleeding caused by heat, cold, excess or deficiency.

Pseudoginseng – invigorates static blood.

Artemisia – helps to warm the womb and stop bleeding.

Herbs Used to Help Build Up the Uterine Lining

If your uterine lining is weak, you have little chance of an egg implanting or surviving. These herbs can help to build a stronger uterine lining needed for a successful pregnancy:

Artemisia – used to warm the uterus and stop bleeding.

Leonurus – used to invigorate uterine blood.

Placenta -- helps to tonify the Kidney Yang.

Red raspberry Leaf – helps to unify the uterus. Dosage: steep in water and drink daily as a tea.

<u>Step Four:</u> Internal Cleansing and Liver Detoxification

Congratulations for getting so far. Now it's time to lay one of the most important foundations for conception by removing toxins from your body by cleansing and re-generating your bowels liver and kidneys. This step involves a 3-day juice cleansing followed by a 7-day parasite cleanse alongside a heavy metal cleanse and a liver detoxification protocol.

Why Cleanse?

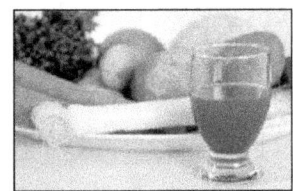

A good cleansing program will not only release you from many disease symptoms (which manifest themselves as chronic pain, hair loss, hormonal disorders, ovarian cysts, and infertility problems), it will give you mental clarity and a serious boost of energy and freedom from many negative thoughts and feelings.

When the digestive system becomes sluggish and over-toxic, it becomes weak and far less efficient. Toxic bowels lead to blood intoxication and a sluggish liver. A weak and sluggish liver that is incapable of handling the over-acidity and toxic overload will release toxins to other parts of the body such as the kidneys, heart, brain, skin, lymph, etc. The result is disease symptoms related to the organ where toxins have chosen to settle. Before any condition such as hormonal problems, ovarian disorders, PCOS or infertility can be permanently overcome, these toxins must be removed.

A deep cleansing program will eventually help the body release toxins from the liver, kidneys and lymphatic system. If followed by a liver purge, it will strengthen and boost the function of these vital organs of elimination, resulting in a more balanced and effective internal system capable of self-healing and handling many infertility related disorders and open your body for conception in the physical and energy levels.

The easiest and cheapest way to cleanse the colon, blood and lymphatic systems is by conducting a series of juice cleansings combined with several detox stimulation techniques.

Cleansing and Infertility

Infertility problems, as well as many other hormonal disorders and illnesses, respond remarkably well to the process of cleansing as eventually most symptoms associated with this condition practically vanish.

The 3-day juice cleansing is a crucial step in the Natural Pregnancy™ System. You will cleanse and rebuild the organs of elimination, help your body expel accumulated toxins and normalize hormone production.

Note: I would strongly recommend combining the juice cleansing session with one of the excellent cleansing kits available here:

Nature's Secret 5-Day Cleanse Kit or HEEL Detox Kit

What Is Fasting?

Fasting is a simple technique where one refrains from consuming any foods or specific types of foods for a certain period of time, which allows the body to recover and heal itself. It's a fact that our bodies have the powerful ability to heal themselves.

When we consume food, our body is busy digesting, processing, analyzing and assimilating. When we go through stressful periods or participate in physical activity, the body is unable to focus on evacuating toxins that have entered and are being stored in our system. When we fast, our body will automatically concentrate its energy on eliminating poisons and cleaning our system; it will recover and heal itself from the various disorders and inflictions it may have.

The principle is simple – we let the body rejuvenate and heal itself through the power of not eating.

Why Should You Fast?

Our body is limited in its ability to evacuate and eliminate vast amounts of accumulated toxic chemicals and foreign materials that were either inhaled, created through stress and anxiety or entered through our system with toxic foods we consumed. These toxic metals and other pollutants are hazardous to our health as they circle the blood stored in our tissues and vital organs. These poisons create a significant burden on our elimination organs such as the intestines, kidneys and liver.

As soon as these toxins enter our system, our body is in fact already in a state of disease. When our body isn't able to handle the amount of toxins circling the blood accumulated in a certain organ, we become sick.

Because a sick person's system is loaded with all kinds of toxins (different types of metals, medication, metabolic waste, etc.), the body searches for emergency ways to discharge itself from these poisons. Often the organ the body chooses to expel its waste through becomes afflicted with symptoms of a disease relevant to its nature.

If the body tries to evacuate poisons from the lungs, you may catch a cold. If it evacuates toxins through your feet, you get athlete's foot. There are various symptoms of overload toxic buildup such as headaches, stuffy nose, allergies, confusion, diarrhea and yeast infection.

The skin is an alternative way for the body to discharge itself from the overload of poisons. It's believed that chronic diseases develop once the body enters a state of extreme intoxication where organs are partly or completely destroyed beyond repair.

Fasting is an excellent solution that relieves the body from stored toxics and allows it to strengthen, heal and fortify itself. Eventually, the fast will clean the bloodstream, cells, tissues and internal organs in general to prepare them for the extreme process of healing.

Types of Fasting

Many types of diets are also referred to as fasts although they aren't particularly so. Fasting in the strict sense of the word is simply avoiding any type of food. In that sense juice cleansing or apple/cucumber cleansing are not fasts but mono-diets.

However, for starters these diets are a great way for new comers to get their feet wet and practically experience fasting. These mono-diets can also function as preliminary stages prior to liver flushing or water fasting but not as a replacement.

With that said, unlike apple or cucumber fasts, juice cleansing is a lot more beneficial. It not only expels accumulated toxins from your body and allows it to rest (Unlike mono-diets, the digestive system rests during liquid fasts), but it also allows more intense cleansing while supporting the body with a variety of nutrients that supply energy and vitality – unlike mono-diets that are limited in their nutrient supply to the certain fruit or vegetable consumed.

That is why I always prefer juice cleansing to mono-diets.

Water fasting is very effective when it comes to healing severe or chronic diseases, yet it's not recommended for inexperienced fasters and cannot be combined with regular daily activities. It's always recommended to start a juice fast plan and "slip" into a water fast to make cleansing and body reactions less intense.

Fasts that are under a week are considered short fasts. While a 1-day fast, if done regularly each week, can strengthen the immune system and credit you with vigor and vitality, 3-day fasts will give your body a real opportunity to "get to work" and make general "arrangements" in your "house." In 3-day fasts (including juice fasts) the body will be grateful as it's given time to thoroughly cleanse your system out of years of accumulated toxic waste.

General Fasting Guidelines

Finding the Time And Place

The ideal time for fasting is a time of relaxation when you are not placed under a lot of pressure or stress or required to invest a lot of energy. That is why a vacation is an excellent and effective time for fasting.

Bear in mind that healing will not happen if you spend your fasting during emotional or mental stress. A fasting period must be a time to save your energies. You must also make sure you fast in a place where there are minimum to no distractions.

Another important factor to consider is the weather. Transaction seasons are best for fasting, whereas fasting in cold weather would be ill-advised as the body temperature in times of fasting is low due to a lack of calories, and it will be easier to get cold when temperatures are low.

I usually conduct my fasting sessions either from Friday till Monday and on the warm holiday seasons.

What To Eat Before The Fast

Fasting is a challenge as you prepare your body for the extreme transition between solid foods and liquids. You must also prepare yourself mentally for the change.

Pre-Juice Cleansing Diet

An effective pre-juice fasting diet would span over a period of at least 3 days before the actual fast. An optimal pre-juice cleansing will consist of salads, juices and fruits. You should avoid consuming refined carbohydrates, bread, dairy products, fish and any kind of meat. It's also important to drink a lot of water.

On the first day of your pre-juice cleansing diet, you should eat cooked vegetables in addition to raw salads, fruits and juices. On the second day you should stick to plain raw salads and raw fruits and drink plenty of juices. On the third day it's recommended that you eat only fruits and juices.

Be sure to follow the guidelines for optimal digestion.

Another option is to have the mono-diets as your pre-fast diets. You can have one day of strictly eating apples and two days of only grapes. You can replace the apples or grapes with sprouts and achieve even greater results as all these types of foods are very effective cleansers.

Fast-Breaking Diet

Our hunger instinct is extremely powerful, and it can be deceiving. Breaking the fast in time, especially longer than 3-day fasts, is an instinct you'll develop as you get more experienced with fasting. It's very important to really feel and know when the time is the optimal time to stop fasting. It's also very hard to guess. You must not only know when to stop, but you must also know how.

Jumping to Burger King and having a Whopper at a time when your liver, kidneys, heart and bowels are in a very sensitive state can cause a stress that may even be fatal. You don't want to stretch the fasting period beyond your needs either. You must control your ego here.

The rule of thumb is to listen to yourself, and listen to your needs. Try to distinguish between a false hunger drive and a real craving for food. The main difference between the two is that hunger is more gradual and starts as mere curiosity with thoughts of food and develops slowly. False hunger is more like a temporary panic attack. This is not

Page 203

hunger; it's your mind fooling you. When you get hungry, you'll know it. Trust me on this.

The gradual craving for food has typical forms such as cheating a little bit and developing a curiosity for food-related subjects, etc. If it's your first long fast, it's recommended to stop the fast at that point.

Followed by the gradual cravings for food is real hunger. When you experience it you'll know. When it comes you must always stop. Otherwise, you're simply starving yourself.

When you break the fast, start by consuming foods rich in water (lemons, limes, cucumbers). Then you can work up to rich protein nut milks. You can start eating soups and plenty of non-starchy vegetables and some whole non gluten grains. 24 hours later you can start eating fats and grains as normal.

Important Guidelines

Eat like a baby in small doses, and eat slowly.

Stimulate the digestive glands by adding celery and clover to your menu.

Broaden your menu with green leaf salads with avocado, tamari and sesame seed dressing (Tahini).

Eat nuts in small quantities only.

You should you broaden your menu only after 2 or 3 days with whole grains and cooked vegetables (broccoli, potatoes, beans).

Tips For A Successful Fast

Take an Epsom salt bath.

Meditate.

Turn off the TV.

Go for walks by yourself.

Close your cell phone.

Limit your conversations with people.

Get a good night's sleep.

Three-Day Juice Cleanse

Introduction

Juice cleanse is a liquid diet consisting of only vegetables, fruit juice, other liquids and water. The juice extracted from raw fruits and vegetables is rich in phytochemicals, alkaline elements, vitamins, minerals, enzymes and natural sugars all absorbed directly into the bloodstream. It requires no effort from the digestive system.

When you do juice cleansing, you mix a lot of different concentrated and powerful fruits and vegetables such as carrots, parsley, celery, green peppers, lemon, etc., into one glass. By doing that you allow the digestion system to easily absorb most of that vegetable/fruit value.

Juice cleansing is much safer and easier than water fasting because it supports the body nutritionally as it gently and safely cleanses and detoxifies it, allowing it to focus entirely on healing itself. Only after you have practically cleansed years of toxic buildup may you take a step forward and start a water fast, which is far more intense.

Juice cleansing operates on two levels. It expels accumulated toxins from your body, and it supports it with a variety of nutrients that supply energy and vitality. Juice cleansing supplies the body with sufficient nutrition and calories, giving you enough energy to go to work, study or whatever. Although you don't really need to change anything in your routine while on a juice cleansing, I recommend that you strive to relax during this time and refrain as much as you can from hard physical activity.

Juice cleansing has freed individuals from most diseases, even chronic diseases such as leukemia, arthritis, high cancer, high blood pressure, liver and kidney disorders, skin infections and infertility and hormonal disorders.

During juice cleansing a lot of metabolic changes occur and a great quantity of toxins are being released from the colon, bladder, liver, kidneys, lungs and skin. The lymph and blood are detoxified. By the third day of your juice cleansing, you'll lose cravings for food, and your digestive system will be in rest, allowing your colon to expel years of disease-causing toxic buildup.

If you find it really hard when on the first 3-day juice cleansing, you may incorporate slices of banana or avocado into your juicing routine, though it's not recommended as it will slow down the healing process.

As for how much you should drink, I can only say drink as much as you please; however, you must minimize acidic and high-sugar fruit juices. They can require the pancreas to produce excessive levels of insulin, which may lead to yeast infection.

One last recommendation: Strive to buy certified organic fruits and vegetables instead of regular ones. Vegetables, especially leafy ones that are not organic contain a high value of pesticides that would also absorb into your system (see also "Cleaning Your Vegetables And Fruits"). Also, make your own juices. By no means should you replace freshly squeezed juices with pasteurized juice or V8 bottled juices.

The Holy Grail Of The Natural Pregnancy™ Juicing

Plan

The only way to maximize the effect of the juice cleansing is by following the guidelines below to the best of your ability.

Consume as many "green" drinks as possible while minimizing fruit and starchy or sugary vegetables. Don't forget wheatgrass.

Drink a lot of water (not tap) and herb teas while minimizing nut milks.

If you must, take only water-soluble vitamins. Take your EFAs and Primal Defense daily, but don't take any minerals.

It's crucial to stimulate the organs of elimination and help them discharge toxins during the fast (liver, kidneys, lungs, intestines and skin).

It's crucial to prevent the re-absorption of toxins into your blood by using daily enemas and drinking bentonite shakes.

Cleaning Your Vegetables And Fruits

Vegetables and fruit that are not organic usually contain high levels of bacteria, pesticides and parasites. Some vegetables and fruit are more available in their organic form than others. For example, it's much easier to find organic carrots in a local supermarket or health food store than to find organic beets or celery.

Agricultural chemicals are hard to get rid of. Some chemicals are even found in organic vegetables. With the proper means and techniques, however, it's possible to clean vegetables from some of their chemicals and parasites.

The most common method is using 4 teaspoons of salt and lemon juice in a sink full of cold water. The vegetables are then soaked with the water and rinsed. You can also put your vegetables in boiling water. It will kill most of the germs, but this method isn't suitable for the more fragile vegetables such as lettuce.

Basic Juice Blends

Fruit Combinations

Watermelon, grapefruit

Apple, watermelon

Apple, pear, pineapple

Apple, grape

Apple, cranberry

Apple, pear

Pear, yam

Watermelon, lemon

Pineapple, sweet potato

Carrot combinations

Carrot, beet

Carrot, beet, green pepper

Carrot, beet, green pepper, parsley

Carrot, cabbage

Carrot, spinach

Carrot, apple, alfalfa sprouts

Carrot, spinach, kale, red pepper

Carrot, celery, cilantro, garlic

Carrot, parsley, cucumber, radish

Carrot, mango

Carrot, apple, ginger

Carrot, celery stick, potato, radish, beet

Warning: Never take beet juice alone. Always mix it with other fruits or vegetables. Beet is a very powerful cleanser, and if taken alone it may cause healing symptoms to become highly intense.

Green combinations

Celery, spinach

Celery, spinach, tomato

Celery, spinach, tomato, cabbage

Celery, spinach, tomato, cabbage, lemon

Celery, spinach, tomato, cabbage, dill, garlic

Celery, spinach, tomato, cabbage, cayenne, dill, ginger

Celery, fennel (anise), cucumber

Tomato, cabbage, garlic, lemon

Lettuce, cabbage, celery, lemon

Lettuce, spinach, cucumber

Lemon, radish, beet, slice of Spanish onion, sweet potato, celery

Note: Green vegetable combinations are excellent nerve tonics, detoxifiers and blood cleansers. One drink of green combination a day will provide you with more than enough.

There is virtually **no limit** on green vegetable juices intake. I usually drink between 1 to 2 liters of green juice daily when I am on a juicing fast.

Wheatgrass – The King Of Greens

Wheatgrass is probably the most powerful juice available on earth. It has tons of chlorophyll, the green pigment found in plants (also called the blood of the plants) that has great healing powers.

Wheatgrass cleans the colon, alkalizes the blood, heals wounds, purges the liver, increases enzyme activity and has lots of vitamin E and antioxidants.

The recommended serving is 2 ounces daily on an empty stomach. Don't drink too much or too soon. It can lead to hyper-detoxification, which can result in nausea.

Other Liquids

Besides juices and water, there are several healthier options to choose from. You can drink herb teas or nut milks, for example.

Herb Teas

Herb teas are made of freshly cut dried herbs known for their culinary and medicinal values. They contain no caffeine and are highly therapeutic. Some herb teas will assist you with nausea and your appetite. Some will supply minerals and vitamins, and some like comfrey are very nutritional. There is almost no limit to how much herb tea you should drink during the fast.

Examples of therapeutic and nutritional herb teas are parsley, peppermint, cloves, alfalfa, comfrey, capsicum, chamomile, rose hips and kelp.

To stimulate digestion use clove, cinnamon, nutmeg.

To stimulate the bowels use licorice, cascara sagrada.

Liver cleansing herbs: dandelion, burdock, yellow dock root (available separately or in the daily detox tea package at: **http://www.amazon.com/DetoxTea**

Rich in magnesium: kelp, parsley, garlic, peppermint

Rich in vitamin C: oregano, comfrey, rose hips, strawberry leaves

Rich in calcium: dandelion, chamomile, kelp

Nut Milks

Nut milks are great appetite breakers, and they are usually good for long fasts (more than 2 weeks) when some people's appetites develop to uncomfortable levels. Almond and sesame milks are very efficient at breaking an appetite for protein. They are good as pre-fast diets, especially for beginners.

Mix these nuts with a teaspoon of honey and a cup of water once in two days only when you're on long juice cleansing and when you start feeling a craving for food. These nut milks are extremely high in protein and fat and are very nutritious.

Avoid cashews as they form a cashew purée (considered a breach of a fast), and their fat may slow down the detoxification process.

Note About Protein and Fasting

Protein exists in every plant on earth. It's nothing but a myth that good sources of protein can only be found in rich protein foods such as meat and cheese. Nut milks as well as wheatgrass powder can be good sources of protein during a fast but should be taken sparingly. In a detoxifying process, protein is not needed. You can practically live without protein for extended periods of time. However, an abnormal craving for rich protein foods during a fast is a dead giveaway that it's time to end the fast.

Apple Cider Vinegar

This is a powerful antiseptic and antibiotic drink. You should buy only raw and unfiltered apple cider made from organic apples only. This drink will act as a powerful cleanser and will help maintain the acid-alkaline balance in your intestines. Add one tablespoon to a glass of water each morning on an empty stomach.

Digestive Enzymes

To improve the breakup of plaque that builds in the bowels, take digestive enzymes on a daily basis. I recommend: Garden of Life Omega Zyme Caplets. Available on the web at **http://www.vitaminsandsuch.com/**

Take the enzymes in the morning accompanied by a slice of fresh ginger with plenty of purified water.

Water

Whatever you do, don't forget water. Water is a powerful cleanser that flushes all kinds of liquids from your bladder and kidneys and digestive tracts. Water is extremely nourishing and also contains lots of valuable minerals.

It's highly important to drink only pure water. No tap water is allowed. These waters are polluted in ways that make it a global problem. Avoid using distilled water also. This water is dead water. Try to avoid drinking spring water, which *is* what it's named after – spring water. It's not pure like most of our lakes and rivers. Stick with filtered or mineral water.

Mixing lemon juice in water also has a laxative effect that stimulates the digestive system. Squeeze half a lemon into warm water. Drink your citrus blend immediately after rising in the morning and before having the bentonite clay and flaxseed shake.

During The Juice Cleanse

What To Look Out For During Juicing

Be on the alert for any allergy symptoms. If you have diabetes or low blood sugar, refrain from sweet juices as you do with sweet foods. These are healing symptoms that may be similar to the symptoms of flu (fever, yeast infection, muscle aches, weakness, bronchitis, asthma). Bear in mind that this is simply the reaction of your body to the vast amount of toxins that now circle your blood stream before they are expelled. Wherever these toxics pass, the organ they're passing through will show the symptoms of that organ-related disease. If they are trying to get out through your lungs, you'll get asthma, through your skin and you'll get rashes and yeast infection. But don't panic. These healing events are short-lived, and the more intense they are, the better your reward is afterwards.

Important note: If your symptoms are truly extreme (for example, if you have a very high fever), it may be time to break the fast. By consuming food, you'll dilute the toxics in your blood stream and feel at ease.

How To Drink Your Juices

Especially when it comes to vegetable and fruit juices, it's highly recommended to "chew" your drink and warm it in your mouth so it will reach your body's temperature. Your juice will get mixed with saliva, which will assist your body in absorbing all the nutrients found in the juice.

Also, leave your vegetables outside your fridge for half an hour before you juice them. It will help the enzymes work even better.

Exercise

Exercise is always advisable. It provides oxygen to the skin cells, and by increasing the flow of blood, it also shortens the healing process of the skin and cleans it from within.

During fasting and a detox diet, it's important to get involved in some exercise activity.

Aerobic exercises such as swimming, walking, jumping on a trampoline and biking are the best because they require an effort from the respiratory system without too much stress and energy. Thus the lungs increase their activity and expel toxins. The lymphatic system also removes waste.

Yoga is another exercise that is very effective in releasing toxins, oxygenating the blood and relieving accumulated tension.

Note: Do not participate in a very extreme physical activity. You must keep in mind that you're on a strict diet, and it can cause fatigue and nausea. This includes running, jogging, weightlifting, etc.

Helping The Organs Of Elimination Remove Toxins

Liver

The liver is an important detoxifier. During a fast it neutralizes and filters toxins coming from other parts of the body as well as expelling its own. However, it's not busy processing newly digested food. This is the time to let the liver rest and clean itself. You can use juices such as wheatgrass, dandelion, parsley, lemon and grapefruit with a tablespoon of olive oil squeezed into some lemon juice to stimulate the gall bladder to release bile.

Cara sagrada and black cohosh are great as cold compresses on the liver and gallbladder.

You can also visit your masseuse and allow him or her to physically manipulate the liver to detoxify and pump the liver slowly and gently to release toxins.

Kidneys

The kidneys have the very important role of purifying the blood and eliminating fluid waste. Drinking a lot of purified water during the fast is a real blessing to the kidneys. There are various herbs that can assist in kidney cleansing and help remove stones (parsley and gravel root, to name a few).

Cranberry, wheatgrass, cucumber and asparagus are also effective kidney cleansers. Taking vitamin C can aid in kidney infections if there are any.

Colon

The colon's main function is to eliminate waste. In fasting there is still waste buildup in the colon pockets, and as they begin to empty, they contain a variety of toxins and acids. Unless these are eliminated, they will be reabsorbed into your colon, resulting in many ill symptoms such as allergies and headaches.

Using enemas, flaxseeds and bentonite shakes will help the colon expel most of its toxins.

Wheatgrass and peppermint act as colon healers, whereas cascara sagrada and mandrake help with the expulsion of toxins.

Juices from apples and carrots serve as great laxatives. Practicing deep breathing may also help to regulate the elimination of toxins and help to heal the colon.

Lungs

The lungs absorb and eliminate a great deal of toxins from the air you breathe. Deep breathing techniques will help the lungs eliminate pollutants much more effectively.

Yoga breathing strategies such as nostril breathing can really aid the process. Drinking alacampange and comfrey herb teas combined with mild aerobic exercise can also help.

Skin

The skin, the largest organ in your body, is where toxins are being expelled all the time. You should treat it with the respect it deserves. While fasting, it's advisable to indulge your skin – brush it, clean it and scrub it to help it expel and eliminate toxins more effectively.

Make sure your skin breathes during fasting by avoiding synthetic clothing. Take short sun baths (Don't burn yourself). Take daily Epsom salt baths and steam baths to accelerate toxic elimination. Rub vitamin E and aloe vera on the skin to prevent dryness.

Keeping A Diary

Good advice while on a fast is to observe your thoughts and feelings during a period without the occupation of eating and digesting. A diary will externalize your deepest feelings, and you'll be able to follow changes in your attitude, notice your weak moments and differentiate between real physical hunger and pure boredom.

You'll be able to observe and educate yourself from your fasting behavior. Note in your diary your interest in food and your anger about not having a "real meal." Usually when real anger attacks you, it's a sign that the fast needs to end.

Vitamin And Mineral Supplements During The Fast

Vitamins and supplements are solid food and thus are a breach in your fast if taken. Besides, you don't need vitamins during a fast as the highly nutritional juices (especially if organic) supply your body with almost everything it needs, and more, for that period of time. Vitamins can also disturb the delicate chemistry balance in your system. The only vitamins you are allowed to take are water-soluble vitamins such as vitamin C.

Preventing Re-Absorption of Toxins Into The Blood Stream

Fiber and Fasting

Taking fiber during fasting can slow down the healing process of the body because it stimulates the digestive system to work. By consuming only juice without fiber during your fast, you allow your system to rest, which intensifies the healing process.

However, without fiber, which is essential for sweeping toxins out of your body, toxins will not be expelled through the colon properly and may reabsorb into the blood. The following methods solve that problem.

Enemas

No matter what negative associations the enema might stir in your mind, doing an enema once a day during a fast is not only compulsory but also very relaxing and even an enjoyable experience once you get used to it.

Enemas are simply meant to rinse your colon with water. Enemas are not intrusive. They are cheap and are done in the comfort of your own home. Enemas are, in a way, an idea of taking responsibility and treating your inside organs with respect. You must help your body discharge accumulated waste that it cannot expel by itself during the fast because there is no bulk of food to help the colon discharge the waste.

One of the reasons why you should pre-fast with raw vegetarian food is that it makes your stool soft and fiber-rich, which is far easier than flushing with water.

There are several types of enemas, I recommend using the water bag enema.

The Process

1) Rinse the enema bag and fill it with lukewarm purified water. A mixture of salt and baking soda can be used to stimulate the immune system. About 1 teaspoon is enough.
2) Hang the bladder about three feet above the floor. This height makes the ideal water pressure.
3) Use a lubricant gel to lubricate the enema tip and anus.
4) You can lay on your side in a comfortable way or simply position yourself on the toilet. However, the optimal position, in my opinion and proven to be the most effective, is simply lying on the bathroom floor head down with your buttocks up.
5) Relax and plant the enema tip fully into the anus and keep a steady flow of water in. It's normal to feel slight cramps; however, if it doesn't feel comfortable, close the tap temporarily, relax and go again.
6) Repeat the process for several times until the enema bag is empty.

Good advice is to massage your abdomen during the process. This will help the enema fluid enter deeply into the colon.

Special Enemas

Depending on your purpose, you can add various mixtures into your enema water to make the procedure more beneficial. For example, you can add wheatgrass to your water, which can be very effective in stimulating the liver to purge itself and can alkalinize the colon. You can add acidophilus to re-establish the friendly bacteria or add vinegar to maintain the proper pH in the colon.

Believe it or not, 2 tablespoons of coffee (organic, fully caffeinated) when taken into the distal sigmoid colon only, can significantly accelerate the detoxification and cleansing of the liver and gallbladder and is especially beneficial before conducting a liver flush.

You can get an enema bag at: **http://www.optimalhealthnetwork.com**.

Psyllium, Flaxseeds And Bentonite Shakes

Psyllium and bentonite are known as excellent colon cleansers. They create a bulk of fluids as they go through the intestinal tract. They absorb and sweep food materials from blocked areas as they move.

Colon cleansers will help you get rid of tons of food debris, which may be accumulated inside your colon. These powders should be consumed with lots of water so it will soften the bulk and prevent it from becoming too hard, which would make it difficult to pass through the intestine.

Bentonite clay and flaxseeds as a mixed shake also aid the colon cleansing process. The bentonite-flaxseed shake acts as a laxative in absorbing and binding toxins, such as pesticides, to form a gel and carry it out of the colon. Flaxseeds alone also absorb water.

How To Make The Shake

Mix one tablespoon of liquid bentonite with one tablespoon of ground flaxseed/psyllium in a glass of water. Take it in the morning immediately so you don't end up with a glass full of gel.

Intestinal Bacteria Replacement

Hormones, antibiotics, drugs and other toxins have a devastating effect on the friendly intestinal bacteria that is so essential in helping the body fight Candida, absorb vital minerals and vitamins, get rid of the toxics accumulated due to constipation and maintain the proper pH in your GI tract.

During fasting, large amounts of toxins are being expelled from the lymph glands that also affect the survival of the beneficial bacteria. The use of an enema also depletes the friendly bacteria.

Therefore, it's mandatory that during fasting, you must make an effort to re-establish the friendly intestinal bacteria. The solution is quite simple. Take 2 capsules of acidophilus and bifidus together with one tablespoon of goat milk yogurt, and mix them together along with a half cup of warm water. Add this blend to the enema kit, and make an effort to keep the mixture inside your colon for at least 10 minutes.

By incorporating this procedure into your daily enema routine, you ensure the friendly bacteria will thrive during your fast.

Warning about Electrolytes

As with beneficial bacteria, you want to ensure that your electrolytes are balanced before and after performing an enema or a liver flush. An electrolyte is a solution or substance that carries electric charges. They exist in the blood as acids, bases, and salts (such as sodium, calcium, potassium, chlorine, magnesium, and bicarbonate). The salts or electrolytes in our bodily fluids allow our nervous system to function properly .

As such, it is imperative to replace the electrolytes after an enema or a liver flush.

This can be done by drinking liquids such as Pedialyte, Gatorade or a glass of water with sea salts.

Choosing a Juicer

When searching for a juicer, besides obvious factors such as quality and price, you must take into consideration another highly important factor. Your juicer of choice must be operated on low speeds so it will not damage the juice by having it absorb too much oxygen, heat up the juice and deplete it of most of its vital fragile nutrients.

While most juicers operate on high speeds from 1,000 to 24,000 rpm's (rounds per minute), low rpm speeds will ensure the preservation of the quality nutrients without destroying the natural flavor of the fruit or vegetable.

A juicer can easily be cleaned and is not limited to juicing only. Certain fruits or vegetables are also important elements you should consider when choosing your juicer.

I found the Omega Model 8003/8005 to be the only cost-effective juicer having all the above qualities and more.

It juices all types of fruits, vegetables, wheatgrass and even other solid foods such as coffee beans, pasta and nut butters. It has built-in "reverse" that prevents clogging, turns at a slow 80 rpm's, prevents heat from building up and is very easy to clean.

You can find out more on the Omega Model 8003/8005 juicer at: **http://www.wheatgrasskit.com.**

Colonics

A colonic is a cleansing procedure where water is introduced through the rectum to clean and flush out toxins from the colon. A typical colonic session may last from forty-five minutes to an hour. This is best done under the supervision of a colon therapist, an expert in colonic. This may also be called a colonic irrigation, colonic hydrotherapy or colon irrigation. The Colonic Procedure After completion and examination of your complete health history checkup and consultation by the hydrotherapist, you wear a hospital gown and lie down, face-up on the treatment table.

The therapist inserts a disposable speculum, which is connected by a long disposable plastic hose to the colon hydrotherapy unit, into your anus. The therapist slowly releases warm and filtered water into the colon. The water causes your colon muscles to contract. This is peristalsis. This causes the feces to be pushed out from your colon through the hose and collected in a closed waste system for disposal .

There could be some discomfort or a weird sensation in the abdomen during the therapy. The therapist massages in and around the abdominal region during the therapy to facilitate the process. The therapist could comment on the color of the feces, although no smell would come out of the closed system. After the session, you may use the toilet to pass any residual water and stools.

Side Effects

Common side effects of a colonic may include nausea and fatigue for several hours. There may be a risk of perforation of the abdominal wall. Careful monitoring is required to reduce the possibility of complications like electrolyte imbalance and heart failure due to excessive absorption of water.

People that should NOT have Colonics

People that have or are being checked for specific medical conditions like ulcerative colitis, diverticular disease, Crohn's disease, blood vessel disease, severe hemorrhoids, heart disease, congestive heart failure, gastrointestinal cancer, abdominal hernia, severe anemia, or intestinal tumors should not have a colonic. You should refrain from having a colonic if you have undergone any recent surgery of the colon. Pregnant women should not have a colonic as it could stimulate uterine contractions. Preparation for a Colonic Before the colonic, drink plenty of fluids and eat only lightly.

After a Colonic

After the colonic, eat very light foods. I also recommend that you eat probiotic foods to restore the good bacteria in your gut. Avoid raw vegetables for few days.

The Healing Crisis and How to Survive It

Every mild cleansing phase such as altering your diet and taking herbal supplements or extreme sessions such the parasite cleanse, 3 day juicing or the liver detox, can and may trigger a healing crisis in which detoxing or die off symptoms manifest. The healing crisis is a natural part of the elimination process on the path to healthy pregnancy, when the body works to regenerate itself and expel waste products through all elimination channels.

When bacteria or parasites die during the cleaning process, these microorganisms release toxins and ammonia. The liver releases stored toxins into the blood stream that also promote familiar healing crisis symptoms.

The more intense the cleanse the faster toxins are released into the bloodstream and the worse you are going to feel.

Here are the most common detoxification related symptoms: Headaches, fever, whiteheads and acne cysts, diarrhea, weakness, irritability, mental depression and nausea.

What you must realize is that once you start improving your diet and lifestyle and begin any detoxification process, **things are naturally bound to get worse before your condition gets better.**

The intensity of the detoxing symptoms as well as the healing process depend on several individual factors: your skin type, your general health condition, your previous lifestyle, the condition of your elimination organs, how much toxins are stored in your system, your energy levels, allergy to certain foods and how effectively your body reacts to the program.

There are in fact several stages for detoxing in which toxins are being expelled gradually and in different levels from your system.

There are also three stages of healing you want to become aware of: At first the body starts to clean up, and rebuild the vital internal organs. This stage depletes energy from your body, which can lead to feeling weak and tired.

My advice is that you sleep and rest as much as possible throughout this stage. The second phase is catabolism: the body starts removing waste material, undigested food, chemicals and hormone residues and releases them into the bloodstream and lymphatic system. During this phase your condition may get worse and you also start experiencing the familiar detoxing symptoms discussed above. Gradually these symptoms will abate and your condition will slowly improve. The final stage is anabolism: the body starts building new tissues and replacing old tissues. This usually causes your energy levels to increase significantly.

The two most important rules during detoxification are: to rest as much as possible during the 3 stages (this will accelerate the healing process) and to accept the detoxification process as a natural part of healing. Be happy with it. Embrace it.

While recovery time varies from one person to another (since it depends on numerous individual factors), it usually takes approx 8-16 weeks for the healing crisis to end and for the detoxing symptoms to abate.

Getting Rid Of Parasites –
A One-Week Program

No cleansing protocol is complete without killing the parasites that inhabit your system.

Parasites are living organisms that eat, lay eggs and secrete toxins into your blood stream. They live off the food you supply them with (especially sugar). They grow healthy and fat and may remain in your body for decades without you even knowing it.

These parasites reproduce inside your body, feeding themselves from minerals like calcium. They eat essential protein and damage your lungs, joints, nervous system and liver. This results in many illnesses such as severe allergies, arthritis, anemia, digestive problems, hormonal disorders, infertility issues and more.

Some parasites can grow up to 15 inches long, inhabit your digestive tract and secrete toxins that create toxic overload.

The most effective and natural way I have found to eradicate parasites is by taking wormwood, cloves, black walnut and garlic herbs daily for the whole week. This will kill most parasites.

Note: as parasites secrete ammonia (which is a powerful toxic), you might feel slightly ill in the process, but don't panic. It's only temporary.

An excellent black walnut and wormwood tincture is available at: **http://www.vitacost.com.**

Note: Start small; take about 5 to 10 drops of black walnut tincture in water. Take a few capsules of wormwood, and a few capsules of ground cloves. Take them all on an empty stomach 2 to 3 times a day. Increase the dose a little each day for six days.

Other good alternatives for killing parasites are consuming plenty of raw garlic. Just be careful. Garlic can encourage a life of solitude. Raw pumpkin seeds are also a good source and contain fatty acids that help in parasite eradication.

Due to its tremendous nutritional value, **coconut oil** is also highly effective for killing parasites. It should be added to your menu even if you experience no symptoms of parasites.

A good quality extra virgin coconut oil is available at:
http://www.vitaminsandsuch.net.

Liver Detoxification

The liver is a remarkably complex and important organ when it comes to maintaining overall health. This is especially true when it comes to infertility patients. Maintaining a healthy liver by promoting liver detoxification is one of the most crucial factors in the successful overall treatment of infertility.

Since the liver is responsible for the production of physiological substances essential for the immune system, and is also one of the major producers of the lymph and helps removing cellular debris, yeast and viruses from the body (with the help of white blood cells), compromised liver function or liver damage can suppress the immune system and contribute to major hormonal disorders.

Improving liver function and enhancing liver detoxification involves 5 protocols:

1.Following a healthful balanced low-fat diet based on whole grains, beans, nuts, seeds and non-starchy vegetables. This will provide the liver with the essential nutrients it needs, including super foods such as garlic and onions that improve its function, while avoiding foods such as refined carbohydrates, hydrogenated oils, alcohol and saturated fats that compromise the liver.

2.Taking high-potency minerals and vitamins. The minerals and supplements outlined in **Step 2** such as the antioxidants and B vitamins will protect the liver from damage and help with toxic elimination.

3.Fasting. The 3-day juice fasting outlined in **Step 4** will greatly enhance liver detoxification and help remove heavy metals and other toxic compounds.

4. Taking specific supplements to protect the liver. This can be achieved by taking the following:

Silymarin

This is a group of flavonoid compounds extracted from milk thistle. These compounds protect the liver from damage (using their highly potent antioxidant properties) and promote liver detoxification -by preventing the depletion of glutathione and even increasing its content by up to 35% (The greater the content of glutathione in the liver, the greater the liver's ability to detoxify).

Recommended daily dosage: 80mg- 200 mg

Available at: **http://www.amazon.com/Silymarin**

Choline, Betaine and Cysteine (Lipotropic Agents)

These nutrients promote the flow of fat and bile from the liver, improve liver metabolism and function, and enhance liver detoxification.

Recommended daily dosage: 1000mg Choline and 1000mg Cysteine

Available at: **http://www.amazon.com/Lipotropic**

Step Five: Nurturing Your Organs and Enhancing Your Qi Through Acupressure and Qi Gong Exercises

PART A: Acupressure Techniques

A lot has been discussed about the importance of preparing your body for pregnancy. You have learned how to live a healthier lifestyle and even how to use a variety of Chinese Medicine techniques to increase your chances of getting pregnant. Now that you better understand the link between your internal energies and your ability to conceive, it is time to learn how to nurture every organ in your body and enhance your Qi. Two of the best ways to do this is through acupressure and Qi Gong exercises.

Mountain Wisdom to the Rescue

Why are acupressure and Qi Gong exercises so important in achieving conception? The Chinese know that if a woman allows stress to overcome her, it will tense her abdomen (the center of her internal energy), and her Qi will be redirected away form the reproductive organs. This can have a devastating effect on her ability to conceive a baby.

For centuries, Chinese medicine has been based on what the Taoists call "Mountain Wisdom." This simple philosophy comes from an ancient story in which an old age from the mountains instructs a young man to empty his cup to make room for the knowledge he had to impart. The younger man refused, holding onto his stresses and burdens, therefore never experiencing the freedom that comes with true knowledge.

Today, that same philosophy reigns within the Eastern medical view, as practitioners find ways to empty their patient's cups in order to find the internal cure to whatever ails them.

Acupressure and Qi Gong exercises are two such ways in which this old mountain wisdom is used today. Both acupressure and Qi Gong exercises have been developed over the centuries as a way to redirect that energy and blood flow to the internal organs that need it and to rebalance a woman internally so that her body can be ready to accept and nurture a pregnancy properly.

Step # 1: Open Your Wind Gates

When we talk about your internal weather, we are talking about the "winds" that can get trapped inside your body, thus creating turmoil both physically and emotionally. Chinese Taoists believe that these "winds" signal "bad weather" or some sort of health crisis. That doesn't mean that you will be struck with a horrible disease, but it can mean that your internal organs are so strangled by stormy winds that they are unable to do their jobs properly. This can – and does – include a woman's reproductive system.

One of the most important acupressure techniques you will learn is one that is used to open the wind gates and free the body of this bad weather. This will help to restore a healthy energy and blood flow to the entire body.

Keep in mind that you may feel some tightness or discomfort while applying pressure to certain organs externally. That is simply a sign of congestion within that organ. Be gentle and continue.

One note of caution here: if you are between ovulation and your bleeding time, be sure to only do these acupressure techniques above the navel, and not below. This will ensure that if conception has occurred, you will not disrupt anything.

Begin to open your wind gates by lying on your back. Think of your navel area as a clock, with 12 o'clock resting in the middle of your chest; 3 o'clock at your right kidney; 6 'clock where your bladder and sexual organs are located and 9 o'clock at the right kidney area.

Now, take a deep breath and relax. First, you will be required to loosen your diaphragm. This is done by taking both of your hands and using them to press firmly toward your navel right under the lower left corner of your ribcage. Continue pressing in this direction until your reach the breastbone, then move to the right side of your ribcage and repeat the process. Be sure to inhale through your nose and exhale through your mouth while performing this technique.

Next, move your attention to the area around your navel. Beginning at the 3 o'clock area where the skin of your navel meets your stomach, apply gentle pressure to each point around the clock face until you feel a pulse. Continue to press down using a spiral motion, unless you feel pain or tightness. If so, then reverse the direction of your spiral. After 3-6 breathes, stop spiraling, but continue to apply pressure to the area.

Next, try to mentally direct warmth to that particular organ. Release the pressure on that organ and take a few moments to relax before moving on to the next organ area. Be sure to work in a counter clockwise fashion. When you have rounded the entire clock, be sure to shake out your hands and feet to reinvigorate your body's energy and give your immune system a jolt.

Step # 2: Try a Groin Pulse Acupressure

Both men and women can benefit from this simple acupressure technique. Designed to increase blood and Qi flow to the reproductive organs, it helps women by ensuring that their ovaries get enough vital essence; while men refer to it as "nature's Viagra," able to greatly improve blood flow to the genitals. For best results, both partners should individually perform this technique once or twice a day.

Begin by lying flat on your back with your knees bent and your feet flat on the floor. Place the fingertips of both hands on your pubic bone. Now, slide your fingers toward your thigh until you reach the fold where your leg meets your abdomen. Lightly palpate this area until you find the pulse.

Placing a finger on each pulse, begin applying pressure in a rotating manner. Your goal here is to get the strength and intensity of each pulse to mimic each other. This may require putting more pressure on one than the other. Once you have achieved this, hold pressure for 35 seconds. Release, and then brush your hands gently down the top of your inner thighs.   Don't be alarmed if you feel a warm tingly sensation. That is completely normal.

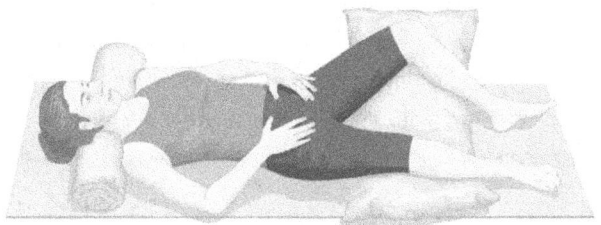

Step # 3: Practice Belly Breathing

In order to completely open your boy's wind gates, it is important to learn to breathe from your belly. This allows you to completely relax, as well as aid digestion and blood flow. Belly breathing isn't hard, but it does take some practice.

Step # 4: The Uterine Lift

A healthy and strong uterus is essential to achieving a healthy pregnancy. Unfortunately, many women are unaware that their uterus may suffer with poor positioning. A lot of things can move your uterus lower in the abdomen than it is supposed to be: childbirth; poor eating habits; even being on your feet too much. Luckily, there is an easy fix with this uterus lift. Using this simple technique, most women can move their uterus back into its perfect position within their body, thus strengthening it for the job ahead.

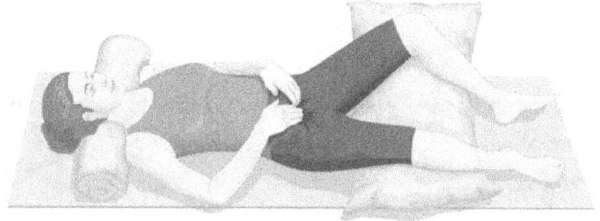

The next time you enter the bathroom to urinate, begin to prepare your uterus for lifting by clenching down to force your urine to pass; than tighten your pelvic floor muscle sin order to stop the flow (this process very much resembles a Kegel). Do this several times during urination.   Now, you are ready to lift your uterus.

Begin by putting your hands on top of your pubic bone. Move your fingertips to a position just above this bone and press hard toward your spine. When you can no longer press toward your spine, you will know that you have reached the area directly under your uterus. Now, use your fingers to gently push your uterus up toward your navel. Hold this position for at least 30 seconds. Release.

PART B: Powerful Qi Gong Exercises

Exercise is the essence of life. If you do not give your body the exercise it needs, your Qi will stagnate, causing serious blockages throughout every organ of your body. Men, especially, can suffer from Qi deficiencies that affect their fertility. So they should take extra care to be sure to stay active.

Of course, not every activity or exercise is good for fertility (for either the male or the female). That is why we are including these important Qi Gong Exercises in this book. Qi Gong is a form of exercise and movement similar to Tai Chai that emphasizes blood and energy circulation throughout the body in order to enhance fertility for both sexes.

Plus, Qi Gong is easier to master than Tai Chai and can also be done in a much smaller space, making it easier for the average couple to do.

Start By Warming Up

If you are interested in incorporating these successful fertility exercises into your daily routine, you will want to begin with a good warm-up. Although the following exercises are best done in the sequence listed, they can be done separately if time is an issue. Be sure to breathe deeply while doing each exercise, and take a moment of rest before moving on to the next one.

Breathing for Energy

Most of us breathe by expanding our abdomen when we inhale and contracting it to exhale. Unfortunately, that is the wrong way to breathe for proper energy flow. Instead try this: contract to inhale and expand to exhale. This is most easily accomplished by breathing fairly quickly (be careful not to get dizzy), while flattening your belly while inhaling. It may feel odd at first, but once you get used to this new way of breathing, you will notice a marked improvement in the energy flow throughout your body.

Laughing

Laughing is a wonderful way to relieve tension, increase your energy and circulation and free your body for the exercises that lay ahead. To laugh for your Qi, try putting your hand on your breastbone, opening your mouth and laughing as hard as you can. Repeat three times.

Next, place your hands on both sides of your ribcage, concentrating on your stomach area. Take a deep breath; expand your ribcage; and then laugh – with your mouth closed – while exhaling. Repeat three times.

Now, concentrate on your lower abdomen, or pelvic area. Take a deep breath and laugh internally, allowing your belly to jiggle a bit, as you exhale. Repeat three times.

Finally, bring your laughing energy to your navel, repeating the above process while concentrating on laughing with your navel.

Loosen Your Waist

End your warm-up by loosening your waist. Begin this process by standing a bit further than a shoulder width part with your feet parallel to one another. Now, turn your hips from side to side with your arms swinging naturally with the motion. After doing this about a dozen times, allow your lumbar vertebrae to begin moving with the motion also. Once you are comfortable with this movement, add your spine, upper back and neck to join in. Be sure to keep your shoulders and arms loose. Repeat several dozen times.

Begin By Opening the Door of Life to Your Fertility

Once you have warmed up properly, you can begin the actual Qi Gong exercises designed to enhance your fertility. Begin by Opening the Door of Life to your reproductive organs. This is done by following the steps below:

Start in the same position as you would for the waist loosening warm-up described above. Only this time, swing your right arm across your front as you move, bringing it up to your head, with the palm facing away. Now, bring your left arm around and press on the Door of Life point on the spine which is found opposite of your navel.

As you reach your full extension, relax, and then extend again, being careful to extend form the Door of Life and not your shoulders. Repeat three times.

Twist to the right, repeating the above steps on this side at least 9 times.

Once you have mastered this basic Qi Gong exercise, try a few of these others:

Tan Tien Hitting

While this is a great fertility enhancer, it is important not to perform the Tan Tien Hitting after ovulation since it could inhibit the implantation of a fertilized egg. That said, feel free to perform this exercise in the first half of your cycle (between the first day of your period and up to 24 hours before you ovulate). Here is how to do it:

Relax your arms completely swinging them in a natural free fall position from left to right until your right hand smacks your navel area at the same moment your left hand smacks against your Door of Life of the back of your spine.
Repeat 35 times on each side.

Knee Rotation

To complete a proper knee rotation be sure to:

Hold your feet together with knees bent.
Place your palms lightly on your knees.
Rotate your knees to the left – gently now!
Now, rotate them to the back and to the right. Repeat 8-10 times
Reverse direction and repeat the entire process

Opening the Spinal Joint

To open all of your spinal joints, you must follow the following 5-phase process very carefully and slowly.

Phase One: Stretching Your Outer Front

Begin this exercise by taking a Waist Loosening stance. Bring your hands together in the front, clasping your hands together. Next, bring your arms around the front and upward until your hands are over your head in a reverse position. Stretch forward, bringing your head down. Slowly continue to bend downward as you feel each lumbar vertebra in your spine release. Slowly stand upright, feeling those spinal joints opening.

Phase Two: Stretching Your Inner Front

Now do the same exercise as above, only in reverse. This will require keeping your hands in an outward position while lowering your back and head.

Phase Three: Bending Your Left Side

For this stretch, keep your arms in an overhead position, than slowly lean and stretch to the left as you lower your arms and head to that side. Continue with this stretch as you bring your arms up and around. Repeat several times.

Phase Four: Bending Your Right Side

Again, repeat the steps above, only in the opposite position in order to stretch the right side of your body.

Phase Five: Finishing Up

To finish opening your spinal joints, unlock your hands and let your arms dangle at your sides.

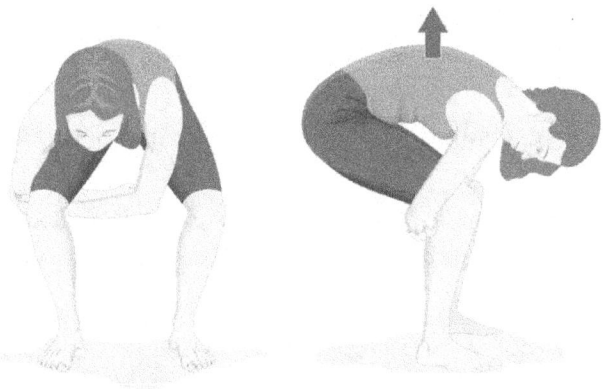

Sidebar: The Three Part Secret to Conceiving a Healthy Fetus: Ovulation, Sperm Count and Sexual Positions/Timing

It takes three vital things to get pregnant and give birth to a healthy baby:

1: Ovulation: Use Fresh Eggs and Sperm

Old ingredients can ruin any recipe – including making a baby! Producing a healthy fetus requires a freshly released egg and sperm. This means abstaining from sex for a few days before ovulation. Remember, a man's sperm can survive up to three days inside of the woman's body; and a three-day old sperm may be defective. Likewise, you should avoid sex right after ovulation, when the egg is still viable but may have aged too much to be healthy. Instead, figure out your peak fertile time for lovemaking, so that a fresh sperm can meet a fresh egg. The best way to do this is to have sex the day before you ovulate.

Of course, determining the exact moment (or close to it) that you ovulate can go a long way to ensuring the egg and sperm are indeed "fresh." One of the best ways to determine the time of ovulation is by using your Basal Body Temperature as a guide.

When you ovulate, your body produces more progesterone, which raises your basal body temperature (usually by about 1 degree F). Of course, this temperature rises up to three days before you ovulate, so while it is a good indicator that ovulation has either already occurred (or is about to), it should only be used as an indicator.

When tracking your Basal Body Temperature make certain to follow these basic guidelines:

Shake down the thermometer before going to bed and leave it on your nightstand to eliminate movement in the morning.

Take your temperature as soon as you wake up before you move, get out of bed, go to the bathroom – any movement at all can alter the results.

Use a basal body temperature for best results.

Take your temperature about the same time every day.

Chart your temperature daily, watching for slight increases that last at least three days. Of course, some women experience an obvious spike in temperature at ovulation (see more on this in the section about BBT).

Note: Increasing cervical mucus can go a long way to helping your partner's sperm make it to it intended target during ovulation. Here are a few simple things you can do to increase your cervical mucus around ovulation time and help increase your chances of getting pregnant:

Take Robitussin Cough Syrup -- taking two teaspoons three times a day with water about five days before ovulation and continuing through ovulation. This has been shown to help loosen the mucus in the cervix. Just be sure that the brand you use does not contain any ingredients other than guaifenesin!

Drink at least 6-8 glasses of water a day to prevent dehydration.

Get enough Vitamin A in the form of Beta Carotene – this helps to improve cervical mucus.

Drink grapefruit juice – to increase the amount of cervical fluid.

Eat plenty of garlic – it helps to thin mucus, both in the lungs and cervical fluid.

Use Evening Primrose Oil to increase production of cervical fluid.

#2: Sperm Count: Build it Up

Prior to Conception

There are a variety of things a man can do to build up his sperm count prior to ovulation to ensure the best delivery possible at baby-making time. For men, this means 3-5 days of abstinence (with no ejaculation at all). During this time it is recommended to participate in some ancient yoga exercises or Tantric Sex practices that can help build up sperm count even further. Participating in several sessions of extended foreplay, but with no ejaculation, can build up sperm levels as well as sperm quality.

Of course, building up that sperm count at the wrong time of the month won't do you any good if your goal is to make a baby. While it is possible to begin building sperm count and motility right away, it's important to begin building sperm counts 3-5 days prior to suspected ovulation. A great way to do this is by practicing oral sex, in which the man is brought close to ejaculation several times before intercourse over a period of about one hour prior to vaginal ejaculation.

#3: Sexual Positions and Timing

Having sex at the right time is essential to getting pregnant. By now you know the importance of having sex just prior to and at ovulation time, but what if you ovulate late? Like after day 16? Then you may find it difficult to maintain a pregnancy even if you are lucky enough to conceive.

Avoid trying to conceive if ovulation

occurs after Day 16

Some cycles are a recipe for disaster, and even if you do manage to conceive, they will likely result in a miscarriage. Cycles with an ovulation time after day 16 is one of them. Why? Because the uterine lining is no longer optimal for nourishing a fetus. If you find that you regularly ovulate after day 16, be sure to tell your doctor!

Does Position Really Matter?

While not everyone agrees that certain sexual positions may increase your chance of conception, many others insist that a standard man on top position will allow gravity to help the sperm along its journey and keep it from resting in the cervix too long. Many couples opt to help nature along even more by using a pillow beneath the woman hips to offer an even greater gravitational pull.

Chapter Five

What to Do During the Program

You've been bombarded with a lot of information thus far, and may be feeling a bit overwhelmed. The odds are, you have already found several new things to try to help you get pregnant, but there are a few important things to remember while incorporating the ideas and suggestions found in this book.

Reading Your Body's Signals and Signs

First and foremost, it is essential that you learn to read your body's individual signals. Your body has the tendency to tell you exactly what it's up to – if you're smart enough to listen. You've heard the stories of women who, after only trying a month or two to get pregnant, instinctively know that something is amiss only to be told by their doctors to keep trying. Finally after a year or more of disappointment their doctor agrees that something is indeed is "wrong" and decides to begin a lengthy testing cycle to determine the cause of her infertility. If only the doctor had listened to the women's instincts right away, she and her spouse could have been saved months of disappointment.

If there has ever been a time for you to listen to what your body is telling you, it is now. The first step is to watch for signs of ovulation so that you ensure the proper response (having sex at the right time). This can be done by watching for important signs such as:

Tender breasts, headaches, mood swings.
An increase in cervical mucus and its elasticity.
A sudden basil body temperature increase of at least .2 degrees that lasts about three days.
Sharp sudden pain in the abdomen.

Keeping a Fertility Chart

Once you have learned how to detect ovulation, you will need to keep a chart of these signs/symptoms in order to *predict* it from month to month.

While it may sound complicated (and often looks that way in the books you read), a fertility chart can be as simple or complex as you make it. Basically, it's just a record of what's going on in your body, with symptoms listed on a piece of paper by your bed, or on an intricate graph on the computer. That's up to you. The important thing is to record your symptoms from month to month so you can see any patterns that emerge which will help you better predict your peak fertility times.

Kits, Sticks and Software That Can Help You Predict Ovulation Better

For some people, predicting ovulation on their own requires the use of more sophisticated methods such as ovulation kits and sticks or even computer software. Others simply want to double-check their own results with these more techno-reliant options.

Using Ovulation Predictor Kits

Ovulation predictor kits are available in most drugstores, and although pricey can be fairly accurate in predicting ovulation in most women. They work by measuring the amount of LH (luteinizing hormone) found in your urine. Since LH generally rises 24 to 36 hours before ovulation, these tests can help you determine about what day you are apt to ovulate from month to month.

There are some drawbacks to these tests however. First, women with polycystic ovaries may have a high LH all the time, so the kits will always be positive, as could women over 40 or those in premature ovarian failure (POF).

They can also be difficult to read and understand so many women must use them for several months for a solid reading.

Using a Spit Test

One of the newest ways to test for ovulation requires you to take samples of your spit. Believe it or not, your saliva's salt content rises as you your estrogen levels increase, so finding your saliva's peak salt line can be a good way to determine when you ovulate.

According to the FDA, these spit tests are about 98% accurate and easy to use. Since you can reuse the testing tubes, the kits must only be purchased once, unlike other ovulation kits which must require buying a new kit every month. Plus, you can use the testing kit anytime, not just when your bladder is full or in the early morning.

Although more expensive (about $60) and harder to use, the salvia test does appear to be more accurate, especially for women who do not have a regular period.

Testing Sperm at Home

Women aren't the only ones who can test their fertility at home – now men can too! Although not as comprehensive and accurate as a formal sperm test, a home semen test can at least give you an idea if the man's sperm count is an issue.

Fertility Monitors

For those wishing to use a more high-tech method of determining their ability to conceive, a fertility monitor may be the answer. Using a small computer to track and store data regarding your test results, these monitors can actually test both your estrogen and LH levels from day to day. Able to predict ovulation five days before it happens, they can give couples a much better chance at success.

Fertility monitors can also be used if you're taking fertility drugs, and unlike other testing kits, it can also be set for women with unpredictable cycles.

They are expensive — running over $200 — but are the most accurate home testing service available.

Getting Through That Two-Week Wait

Waiting can be hell – especially when you're every hope and dream hinges on whether or not you've managed to get pregnant. Since you can not accurately predict a pregnancy until at least two weeks after conception, most couples become a basket case during this short waiting period. So how can you get through it without upsetting your internal balance and driving yourself (and each other) nuts?

 Here are a few suggestions:

Get busy with a new project. Nothing takes your mind off of any issue – including whether or not you're pregnant – like diving headlong into a new project.

Avoid thinking (and talking) about babies during this time of the month. I know that it's hard, but try. Constantly letting your mind wander back to babies and pregnancies will only make the wait seem longer.

Have some fun. Go on vacation. Visit family and friends. Go to the theatre. Choose an activity to enjoy that you know you won't be able to do for awhile once you do indeed conceive a child.

Have sex just because you want to. For many couples trying to conceive, sex becomes more of a chore than an enjoyment. Have fun again! Enjoy each other. Consider this: once you become parents, you'll have a lot less time and energy for sex so you'd better have some fun now.

The Importance of Exercising Correctly

Exercise has many benefits for both men and women trying to conceive including strengthening their body; oxygenating tissues, cleansing toxins and alleviating the stresses that could all be inhibiting conception. Of course too much exercise can also be a detriment, causing depletion in the Yin and estrogen in the body. Focusing too much energy on the skeletal system can take important energy from the reproductive system, so be sure to be smart about any exercise routine you undertake. Too much is just as bad as too little.

Control Stress

Chances are you have heard this advice during your quest to have a baby: just relax. Easier said than done, but the fact remains: stress can be a major road block on the journey toward parenthood.

Referred to as the "fertility killer" stress can impact the way our bodies both act and react. Putting your body into a fight or flight response with too much stress, can inhibit the reproductive system from doing its job. Stress redirects blood flow away from the areas you need it most in order to conceive. This can keep your body from producing the right amounts of hormones or even going through each phase of menstruation on time or in the right order. Remember, just one little part of the system out of whack and the entire system can fail!

A recent study at the University of California concluded that women undergoing gamete intrafallopian transfer (GIFT) a highly technical fertility treatment were 93% more likely to achieve a pregnancy and live birth if they exhibited little or no signs of undo stress going into the procedure.

The Chinese don't have a word for stress in their vocabulary. They call this phenomenon Liver Qi Stagnation, which they say is caused by unfulfilled desires. Considering that failing to conceive may be a human's most intense failure to fulfill their desires, it's no wonder that stress can affect a couple's ability to have a baby. Doing your best to alleviate stress can be a big benefit to getting pregnant, especially if used in conjunction with other therapies.

Sleep Optimization

We all know how important sleep is to our health, but what about to our fertility? Your body can't reach its perfect balance without the right amount of sleep. Be sure to get at least eight hours of solid sleep each night and be sure to take time throughout the day to relax rest and meditate in order to keep your body in perfect harmony.

Femoral Massage

Adding Femoral Massage to your diet and exercise routine is known to increase blood flow to the pelvic organs, which provides even more nourishment to the ovaries and uterus. To perform femoral massage to your pelvic region, follow these steps (they may be easier with a partner):

Step I: Using your fingertips, apply pressure to the large artery beneath the crease in your groin (between the thigh and lower abdomen). This is your femoral artery. It comes from the iliac artery which supplies blood to the uterus, fallopian tubes and ovaries and the kidneys.

Step II: Press on the artery until you feel the pulsation stop. Hold for 30-45 seconds. This will cause the blood to stop flowing, backup into the iliac artery, forcing more blood into the pelvic organs.

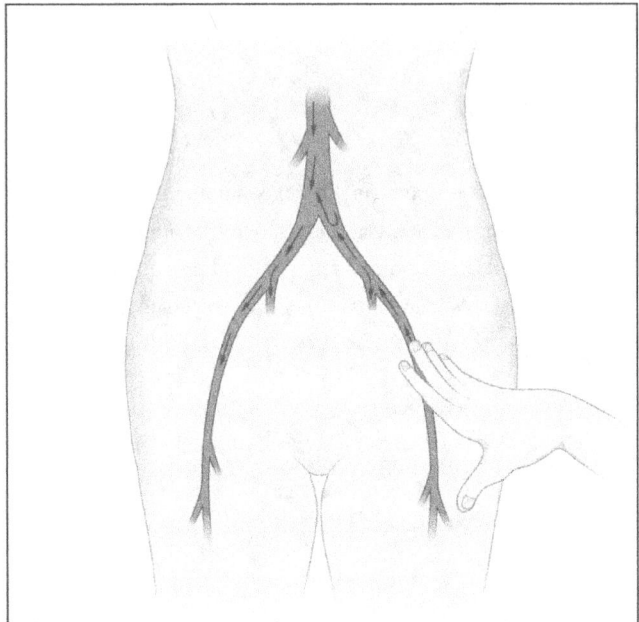

Figure 6: Femoral Massage

Step III: Release the pressure in less than 45 seconds to allow normal blood flow once again. Don't be surprised if you feel a warming sensation down your leg when the pressure is released. This is just your blood rushing through the artery to your lower extremities.

Step IV: Repeat on the opposite side. Then repeat the entire sequence three times in a row, twice a day until ovulation day.

SPECIAL NOTE: Do not perform this exercise if you are or may be pregnant, have high blood pressure, heart disease or any type of circulatory problems, detached retinas or are at risk for a stroke!

Qi Gong Breathing

The Chinese believe that using this breathing exercise can literally "breathe life in and through the uterus." To practice Qi Gong breathing, do the following:

Place the tip of your tongue on the roof of your mouth, just behind the top front teeth.

Breathe in deeply through your nose, concentrating on moving the breathe from your nose; down the midline of your body; between the breast; through the abdomen; and down into he region about two inches below the navel. Let he breathe energy pool here, pushing out on your belly as you inhale.

As the inhale ends, move your focus from the area below your navel to your uterus and the muscles of your vagina. Next, do a kegel exercise by squeezing your pelvic floor muscles as if you were trying to stop your urine from flowing.

Release and exhale, while changing your focus up the spine into your head, then down the midline of the head and out of your nose.

Repeat steps 2, 3 and 4 until they become a more natural, singular movement.

This exercise can be done as often as you like, except when you are menstruating or pregnant.

Male Infertility Plan: The 4 Step Program to Tackling Male Infertility Factors – Low Sperm Count and Motility and Low Testosterone Levels

In the vast majority of low sperm count and motility and low testosterone cases the following 4 steps have been tested and proven to help produce healthy sperm and dramatically enhance sperm motility, therefore reversing most male infertility issues:

Male Infertility Plan -Step 1: Dietary Changes

Increase the daily dosage of the following foods:

Red meat - pork, beef, lamb (organic or hormone free)

Fish - preferably oily fish such as salmon, trout, tuna (organic)

Eggs and vegetarian dairy substitutes

Beans and legumes - kidney beans (soak in water for the night prior to cooking)

Leafy green vegetables and cruciferous vegetables such
as broccoli and cauliflower– preferably organic

EFAs and Vegetarian sources of EFAs - avocados, brazil nuts, pumpkin seeds

Fresh fruit and vegetables – preferably organic

Try to avoid the following foods/habits:

Foods which contain caffeine such as coffee, tea, chocolate.

Processed canned and fabricated foods. This includes all artificial ingredients,
additives, food coloring and food additives.

Industrial non organic meat

Fried foods.

Eating in excess.

Male Infertility Plan -Step 2: Supplements and Herbal Remedies

Take the following supplements and herbal remedies on a daily basis for a period of 8-12 weeks to help increase sperm count and motility:

1. Vitamin A – 3000-10000 IU

2. Vitamin B – 1000-1,500 mcg daily (or B Complex)

3. Vitamin C – 1000 mg daily

4. Vitamin E - 400 mg daily

5. Zinc – 10-50 mg daily

6. Selenium - 100 mcg

7. Arginine - 5 grams, 30-45 minutes before sexual intercourse

8. Carnitine - 3 grams a day

9. Maca Root in powder form

10. Sarsaparilla (1-2 grams twice a day).

11.Chinese Panax Ginseng -Take 200mg to 600 mg a day – this herb helps not only with sperm count and motility problems it can also help with erectile dysfunction.

Note: make sure all supplements you take are from natural preferably organic sources and not from synthetic sources as most of these are practically useless.

Male Infertility Plan -Step 3: TCM and Chinese Remedies

Traditional Chinese Medicine can dramatically help you balance your energies, enhance your reproductive system and improve sperm count and motility.

Simply hold the following acupressure points for a minute or so twice a day for several weeks: Kidney 7 and Lung 8 at the same time, and Spleen 2 and Circulation Sex 8 at the same time.

Also, massage points Stomach 36 and Bladder 66 for 1 minute twice a day.

The following Chinese herbal remedies can also help improve poor morphology, sperm count and motility and increase testosterone levels:

Blood and Qi tonics along with seeds such as and Cuscuta

Qi tonics containing ginseng (ren Shen)

Cornus (Shan Zhu Yu).

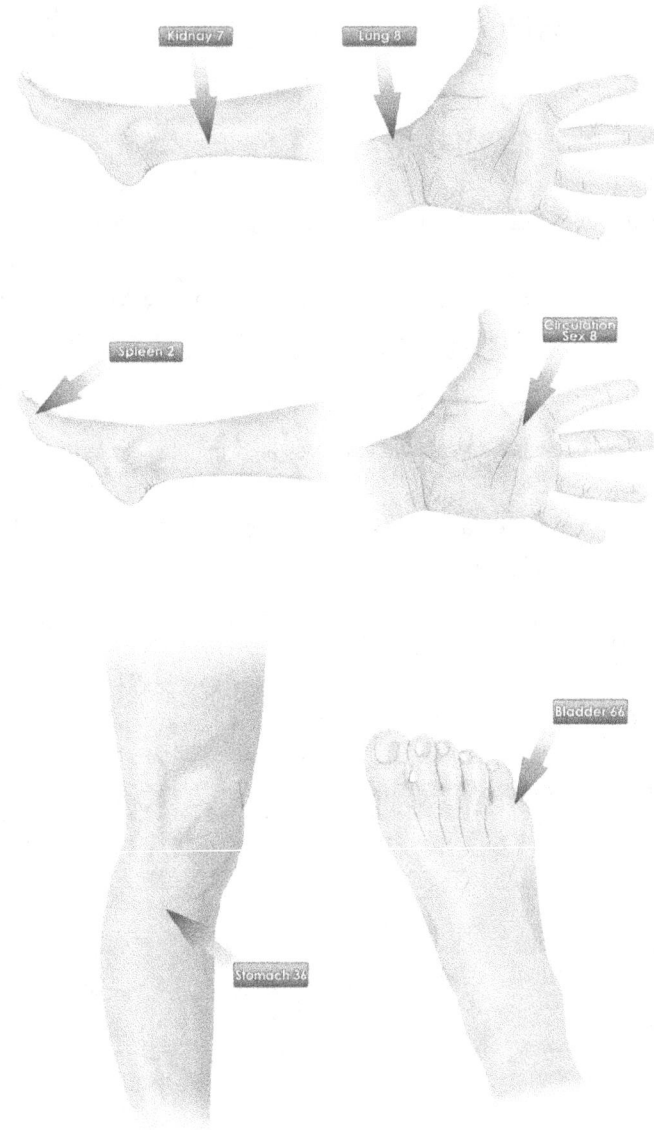

Male Infertility Plan -Step 4: Lifestyle Changes

There are quite a few cases where men had completely eliminated their sperm count or motility problems simply by incorporating the following lifestyle changes:

Avoiding stressful situations. Learn how to control or reduce stress and anger.

Reduce alcohol consumption and stop smoking

Stop taking conventional medication – consult your doctor

Incorporate plenty of organic fruit and low starch vegetables into your diet.

Switch all household goods and cosmetics to eco-friendly equivalents

Avoid putting your laptop computer on your lap

Keep your testicles cool - wear boxers, avoid warm environments such as saunas and avoid wearing tight clothing.

Chapter Six

Special Conditions and Other Infertility Related Disorders

Page 270

For some of you reading this book, there are special, more unique problems to be faced. Maybe your infertility stems from advancing age; endometriosis; or even prior cancers. Under these circumstances, you may need to consider additional treatment options. In order to determine what other traditional and non-traditional treatment options you need to consider, we must first take a look at some of the unique issues you may be facing:

Immune System Problems

Immunological issues can affect fertility in two ways:

1. by causing an autoimmune reaction in the body
2. by creating antisperm antibodies which attack and kill off sperm

Autoimmune Reactions

Autoimmune issues may account for 20% or more of infertility issues and recurrent miscarriage rates. With more and more women suffering of late with autoimmune disorders like allergies, lupus, Crohn's Disease, Rheumatoid Arthritis and thyroid issues, it is no wonder that immune system malfunctions account for so many fertility problems.

To detect autoimmune deficiency have your doctor check these four main markers:

1. antithyroid antibiotics

2. antiphospholid antibodies

3. natural killer cells

4. antinuclear antibodies

Anti-thyroid Antibodies

Low thyroid levels, otherwise called Hypothyroidism, is usually caused by high levels of antibodies that attack the thyroid glands. This can keep them from working properly to release the proper se hormones at the right time, thus inhibiting pregnancy. Worse yet, these anti-thyroid antibodies can also induce a miscarriage if they cross-react against the placenta after conception.

Anti-phosphotipid Antibodies (APA's)

When APA's are present in the bloodstream, they attack normal cells, believing them to be nasty invaders wanting to do the body harm. When this happens they attach themselves to fat molecules of the cell membranes, creating clot. This keeps blood from flowing to the endometrium, which will ultimately keep an egg from implanting in the uterus.

One of the best treatments for APA is low dose aspirin therapy. More serious cases may requires anticoagulants to thin out the blood and improve circulation to the uterus. Acupuncture to can also help to improve blood flow. It can be used alone, or in conjunction with the other therapies discussed.

Natural Killer Cells

The immune system needs the very aggressive white blood cells called natural killer cells in order to seek out and destroy dangerous bacteria and viruses that invade the body. Even cancer cells can be destroyed natural by these killer cells before they have a chance to multiply.

There job doesn't stop there, however. Natural killer cells are also found in the uterine lining where they help to aid implantation of the fertilized egg. Problems can arise though if these natural killer cells go into overdrive and begin to attack the embryo instead of help it.

Once a blood test indicates that natural killer cells are present in abundance, then a treatment of intravenous gamma globulin, steroids or intralipid infusions are given to help suppress this dangerous immune system response.

Antinuclear Antibodies

Antinuclear Antibodies are common infections in the body that exist to attack invaders that can make you sick. The problem is, when too many Antinuclear Antibodies are present, they can cause inflammation in the uterus and keep implantation from taking place.

Should high levels of Antinuclear Antibodies exist, steroid treatment id often prescribed. While many people may think that boosting the immune system may help to keep these AA's under control, the opposite is actually true. Instead of super-charging the immune system, the key to controlling Antinuclear Antibodies is to simply bring it back into balance. This is done by using circulation-boosting herbs; increasing your antioxidant intake; reducing stress; taking zinc supplements; and eating more alkaline producing foods like whole grains and fresh organic vegetables.

Antisperm Antibodies

The #1 immune system issue that affects a couple's fertility is an allergic reaction to sperm. When anti-sperm antibodies are present in the female partner's body, they can kill off the male partners sperm – stopping any chance they have at conception.

But, it isn't always Antisperm antibodies in the woman's body causing fertility chaos; sometimes the man's own body can make antibodies that kill off his sperm or make them too weak to penetrate the egg.

Since anti-sperm antibodies can be hard to detect, checking for dead or shaking sperm in the presence of healthy cervical mucus may indicate an antisperm antibody issue. An immunobead binding test can also be performed to look for beading on the sperm after it has been mixed with blood from both partners.

Low dose steroids are usually recommended to help suppress a bad immune reaction when anti-sperm antibodies are present.

When it comes to dealing with immune system breakdowns on your own, here are a few helpful tips:

- meet with a Chinese medical practitioners who has experience dealing with infertility caused by immune system issues in order to devise a treatment plan that meets your specific needs
- begin a yoga and meditation exercise plan to help reduce your stress
- eat plenty of nutritious foods – especially those loaded with healing antioxidants
- stay away from refined sugar and processed foods
- eat more alkaline-based foods
- avoid alcohol
- avoid caffeine
- take a zinc supplement
- get at least 2,000 mcg of folic acid every day
- try the Chinese remedy Zhi Bai (it is great at reducing antisperm antibodies)
- use acupuncture to improve blood flow to the uterus
- take a fish oil supplement daily

As you can see there, are plenty of things that can cause havoc with your fertility, making it difficult to conceive. Hopefully though, you have found that educating yourself on these common fertility issues (and their treatments) is an important first step to discovering a way to break through your own fertility problems and conceive the baby that you have always wanted. Most infertility issues can be handled quite successfully, offering hope to prospective parents. A baby is in your future – sometimes the road to parenthood just takes a few unexpected detours!

Dealing with Advancing Age

Whether we like it or not, we women have a limited reproductive life span. Beginning well before we are ready to be mothers, and often ending well before we are ready to say goodbye to our ability to conceive and carry a child, we are often stuck trying to find the right time in between these two milestones to start or continue our family.

In addition to losing our ability to conceive, many women experience trouble getting pregnant as they age. This is due to a lot of reasons: poor health; stress; older eggs; etc. The fact of the matter is, as we age our bodies begin to get weaker – but only if we let it! If we can eat right and exercise our way to a longer lasting and healthier life, then doesn't it make perfect sense to believe that we can do something (anything) to prolong our fertility – or at least enhance it while we do still have it? Of course it does!

The Chinese believe that a woman's ability to bear children rests in her congenital source of Qi. If it remains strong and in balance, her ovaries will continue to release healthy eggs until they run out. They do not believe that a woman's aging eggs are not able to be fertilized or grow into a healthy embryo; they believe it is the change of her hormones caused by imbalanced Qi that affects the eggs later in her reproductive life. When the hormones are disrupted, it becomes harder and harder – and eventually impossible – for a woman in her 40's and 50's to get pregnant. While a natural progression, time doesn't have to be our enemy. The fact is that your eggs do not have a shelf life as some western medical practitioners would have you believe. As long as you can maintain the right hormones at the right times throughout the month, you can – and will – get pregnant. Treat the two areas affected most by a woman's aging reproductive system (the kidneys and the spleen), and you *can* turn back the hand of time (at least temporarily) and achieve the pregnancy that you desire.

SIDEBAR: A Chinese Look at Aging

Chinese Medicine runs on the philosophy that the three main meridians (the penetrating, conception and governing meridians), are the equivalent of the HPO axis which become fulfilled when a girl begins to menstruate. Since her reproductive age span is a direct result of her underlying Qi energies (both in the Kidney and the Essence), it must be supplemented through the spleen throughout her life to keep her reproductive organs working properly.

The Penetrating Meridian is very important – originating in the uterus and governing over the Yin and the Yang of the endocrine system.

According to Chinese Net Jing, a woman's essence begins to decline when she reaches 49 and her menses cease. This usually happens over many years and is a very smooth and natural progression. Problems arise, however when environmental impacts cause the Net Jing to stop working earlier than the age set by nature, interfering with a woman's fertility.

A woman experiences many changes in her internal energies beginning with an energetic focus at the beginning of menses and flowing from one full moon to the next, eventually transferring energies from the uterus to the heart as her reproductive lifespan comes to a close. This allows the woman to move from a state of procreation (fertility), to a state of wisdom as her fertility abilities cease. If your body becomes resistant to this transition, you may experience an obstructed Qi which can cause hot flashes, mood swings and other side effects.

When TCM is used to stall this transition by re-regulating the hormones needed for conception, you can make the reproductive organs function again – at least for awhile -- and retain a certain amount of youth with higher levels of fertility.

How can this be done? Acupuncture, herbs and the right diet and exercise can all be used to handle deficiencies in the spleen and kidneys and get your body working the way it should in order to get pregnant.

SIDEBAR: Putting age in its (proper) place

Age may affect getting pregnant, but it doesn't have to stop you altogether! Here are a few things that can help you better your odds of conceiving at any age (even an older one):

Get your body in the best baby-making shape as possible -- eat well, get plenty of rest and exercise and see your doctor!
Consult with an OB/GYN or reproductive endocrinologist, experienced in working with older moms. Not all fertility doctors specialize in advanced maternal age, so be sure that yours does.
Get a good support team. Friends, family, clergy and even professional help, can all get you through this trying time.
Consider your options.
Set a timetable. Don't let getting pregnant set you in a tailspin. Think about how long you want to spend trying to have a baby, and stick to it as best you can.
Investigate alternative treatment options.
Be patient. Getting pregnant can take awhile at any age, but the older you get the longer it takes, so be patient.

Infections

One of the most commonly overlooked causes of infertility (in both partners) is infection. As a matter of fact, the vast majority of unexplained infertility cases can be linked back to some sort of infection, with as many as 30% being discovered upon further scrutiny.

To help increase a couple's chance at conception during IVF many doctors are now recommending antibiotic treatment to kill off bacteria in the reproductive tract before undergoing the fertility procedure.

Keep in mind that when we talk about infections here, we are not necessarily talking about Sexually Transmitted Diseases (STD's), or their accompanying bacteria. Although some STD infections do cause fertility issues, the vast majority of fertility-related infections are ire generic in nature.

One common infection women often don't know they have is Chlamydia, which can develop into pelvic inflammatory disease (PID). As discussed earlier, OID can scar the fallopian tubes and impede a pregnancy. Other common infections in the reproductive tract include:

- E-Coli
- Enterococcus
- Staphylococcus

- Ureaplasma

- Mycoplasma

- Candida Albicans (yeast)

Not only can these infections cause damage to female eggs, fallopian tubes, cervix and uterus, but they can also kill off sperm! Female infections can attack sperm causing them to stick together and keep them from making their way to their way to the egg. Sometimes, they attach themselves to the sperm, sucking their energy during the journey, ply to leave the sperm unable to penetrate the hard egg shell once it reaches its destination.

Bacteria in the cervix can also attach itself to the sperm in a way that allows it to reach the egg and penetrate it, only to attack the growing embryo once fertilization takes place. This can result in a miscarriage.

When found, bacterial infections need to be treated in both partners since they've likely transmitted the infection back and forth between themselves during intercourse.

The best course of action in relation to infections is of course preventing them in the first place. This can be done by boosting the immune system with plenty of nutritious foods and immune-building supplements. Garlic too can offer a strong antibacterial properties. Taking antibiotics and probiotics too can help rid the system of dangerous bacteria, while strengthening the good bacteria the body needs within the intestinal tract.

Page 282

Elevated Prolactin Levels

Prolactin is a hormone that helps women to produce milk after the birth of a baby. When levels are high, ovulation is hindered; that is why many nursing mothers do not get a period while their babies are nursing at peak capacity.

Reducing estrogen levels in women and progesterone levels in men, prolactin can have a serious effect on both male and female fertility; causing a loss of ovulation in the female and a poor production of sperm in males. Some common natural remedies for elevated prolactin levels includes:

- taking vitamin B, magnesium and zinc supplements
- reducing stress
- getting enough exercise
- avoiding alcohol
- taking rebalancing hormones such as Chasteberry
- taking qi moving herbs

When it comes to dealing with nay fertility problem, it is important to take as much control over your treatment as possible. Some simple ways that you can help to alleviate elevated prolactin levels include:

1. Add lots of B vitamins nd zinc to your daily diet

2. Avoid alcohol (no amount is safe)

3. Begin a stress relieving regiment including exercise, massage, hypnosis, meditation, yoga, etc.

4. Take a chasteberry supplement to lower prolactin levels

5. Take qi moving herbs

6. Avoid excessive exercise (but gentle exercise is good)

Luteal Phase Defects (LPD)

Many women who cannot get pregnant or who may experience repeated miscarriage often suffer from a luteal phase defect, which simply means that the luteal phase of their cycle (the time between ovulation and their menstrual flow) is too short to develop a thick enough uterine lining to support a fertilized egg. This can either result in an inability for the fertilized egg to implant in the first place, or an inability to thrive, thus resulting in a very early miscarriage. Some women actually miscarry every month without realizing it believing that they are simply having a regular period.

The cause of this disorder is generally low progesterone levels, although low FSH and LH levels can also be to blame. Some signs that you may suffer with a luteal phase defect include:

- Ovulating before day 10 of your cycle or after day 20 (this can be determined by using an ovulation predictor test or charting your basal body temperature and cervical mucus).
- Pre-menstrual spotting
- Menopausal symptoms

When a LPD is suspected, your doctor will likely request one or more of the following tests:

Progesterone Levels – progesterone levels must be scheduled throughout the cycle (typically on days 21, 23 and 25) to see whether or not the progesterone in your body is sufficient.

Prolactin Levels – elevated prolactin levels can cause a decrease in progesterone

Thyroid Function – if the thyroid is not functioning properly it could result in lowered hormone levels or ill-timed hormone release. Thyroid function is usually monitored with a TSH blood test.

Polycystic Ovarian Syndrome – A common disorder among infertile women, PCOS can cause the ovaries to fail to release an egg for fertilization or for release to happen at the wrong time in the cycle. Tests for PCOS usually include a fasting glucose blood test as well as LH and FSH levels.

Once a diagnosis of LPD is made, there are several options for treatment. In many cases fertility drugs such as Clomid are used to boost progesterone levels and make a pregnancy possible.

As the awareness of side effects (including multiple births) of using these drugs is increased, more and more couples are opting for natural methods of fixing LPD. Traditional Chinese Medicine offers some good options for treating this disorder without the use of dangerous drugs.

Chinese Medicine considers LPD to be a whole body imbalance; not just one of the luteal phase of the menstrual cycle. According to Chinese medical practitioners, the luteal phase is governed by Yang energy in the body. It is this yang energy that creates the yin energy which is necessary during the follicular stage of the cycle. The transformation from one type of energy to another (the yang to the yin) is caused by the movement of qi and blood during ovulation. Any disruption of this energy flow can cause LPD. It doesn't matter whether you have too much or too little yin or yang at certain stages or if circulation is bad and the energy cannot move properly, the fact is that if these two energies can not move freely and transform at the fight times of the woman's cycle, a pregnancy is impossible.

Luckily, there are a variety of herbs that can be used in conjunction with acupuncture treatments to help free blocked energies and help balance out yin and yang in order to better balance the hormone levels in the body.

Chasteberry is an excellent herbal choice for treating LPD since it helps to lengthen the luteal phase and hasten the LH surge to ovulation. Recommended dose: 16 drops of tincture twice a day from ovulation to your bleeding time begins.

Red Raspberry Leaf can be used in a soothing tea to help increase blood flow and circulation to the uterus which can help to free blocked energies and increase uterine health.

Acupuncture too is a wonderful treatment for LPD. It is used to free blocked meridians and restore proper energy flow throughout the entire body, with a concentration on the reproductive system. Be sure to find a qualified acupuncture therapist who specializes in treating infertility.

Battling Unexplained Fertility Issues

One of the most terrifying diagnoses a couple can get when trying to find out why they aren't pregnant is "unexplained infertility." The reason is simple: if you don't know what's wrong, you can't do anything to fix it. That can leave many fearing the worst – never having a baby. Unexplained infertility means that there is no definitive medical reason why you shouldn't be conceiving: both of your bodies are working correctly and there are no visual problems for doctors to treat -- so much for medical science.

The fact is there are thousands of reasons why conception could be hindered in any given month: a single hormone isn't produced at the exact moment it is needed; the Ph level of your cervical mucus changes; or even a millimeter less depth in your uterine lining can all play a part in this delicate game. So what do you do when modern medicine has failed to give you either an answer or a baby? Maybe it's time to look at the other methods we've discussed, including Traditional Chinese Medicine (TCM).

The use of TCM may be the most effective in treating unexplained infertility and for good reason: it doesn't rely on fixing a specific symptom, but in treating the entire woman (or some cases the whole couple). The first step, of course, is to review the manifestation of the problem and discover its underlying pattern. Then, and only then, can the practitioner develop a treatment plan.

Treating Secondary Infertility

When people think of an infertile couple, they often envision a husband and wife who for years try to conceive only to be left childless. This isn't always the case. Some couples quite easily conceive their first, second or even third child, only to be left disappointed and frustrated when they try to expand their family. This can be especially difficult when those around them insist that they be happy with the blessings they already have. True, one or two children are a blessing to any family, but they can't take away the heartbreak of being unable to conceive again, or even worse, failed pregnancies following a live birth.

It can be hard to understand why getting pregnant again has become so difficult, but there are many reasons including:

Aging. As we already discussed, you may find it harder to get pregnant as you get older, especially if your hormones are out of whack.

A new partner. In the event you have a new partner this time around, you may face new challenges.

Changes in your health. Any health issues that have arisen between the birth of your last child and your failure to conceive this time around should be considered.

Difficulties with your last pregnancy and/or labor. Any complications you experienced during your last pregnancy and/or labor may have a direct influence on your future ability to conceive.

Stress levels. Being a parent can be stressful. If you find your stress levels much higher now than while trying to conceive your last child, you may need to do something about it.

Diet and Lifestyle changes. Remember, anything and everything can affect your fertility. Do you eat more junk food (and less fresh fruits and veggies) than you did in the past? Are you overweight? Have you stopped exercising? Have you picked up any other bad habits? All of these lifestyle changes may affect your ability to get pregnant.

Physical Reasons Why You May Not Be Getting Pregnant

There are a number of physical ailments which could make it more difficult for you to conceive like: Endometriosis, Fibroids, Ovarian Cancer and more. But that doesn't mean you can't have a baby, you just need to understand your condition and how to treat it for better success.

How to Heal Your Ovaries
Using Chinese Philosophy

Dampness or phlegm is the most common cause of PCOS, with symptoms like:

Sluggishness after meals.

Fibrocystic breasts.

Cystic acne.

Urgent, bright and foul smelling stools.

Mucus-filled menstrual blood.

Vaginal itching (recurrent yeast infections).

Achy joints.

Obesity.

A wet, slimy tongue.

All of these symptoms may be caused by a number of deficiencies which can also affect ovulation. For instance, a Yang Qi deficiency may keep fluids from moving through the body properly. Since your treatment will depend a great deal on your specific diagnostic patterns, here are a few general recommendations for treating PCOS the Chinese way:

Diet Therapy

Most women suffering with **PCOS** have some sort of endocrine abnormality that is affected by their diet. If you are overweight, you can do a lot to treat your PCOS by losing weight since fat cells store estrogen, in which you already have too much. Improper liver function must also be addressed since the liver helps the body metabolize insulin properly. In order to maintain proper insulin balance, try these suggestions:

Stop eating refined sugar.
Avoid refined carbohydrates.
Do not eat a lot of yams.
Avoid all high sugar drinks (soda , fruit juice).
Eat enough protein.
Eat plenty of fresh fruits and vegetables every day.
Eat only whole grains.
Avoid dairy products.
Eliminate caffeine from your diet.
Increase your fiber intake.
Get plenty of exercise.

Herbal Therapy

There are several herbs that are used to treat PCOS:

Gleditsia -- PCOS creates a waxy capsule around the ovaries which can be eliminated by taking Gleditsia (Zao Jaio Ci).
Leonurus Seed – encourages ovulation and is used to treat blood stasis.

Acupuncture Treatment

Studies have shown that one-third of all women suffering with PCOS can find help with acupuncture treatments by reducing the level of hypersympathetic nervous system result and relaxing the endocrine system.   This is done, of course, by restoring balance to the patient's nervous system. This in turn helps to normalize the hormonal response tied to ovulation and reproduction.

Ovarian Cysts

Ovarian cysts are very common fluid-filled sacs inside the ovary. Most of these cysts go away on their own, but some need to removed via laparoscopy. One herbal treatment not available over the counter is a mixture of herbs created by a certified herbalist including Astragals Root, Gleditsia Spine, laminaria, prunella flower, scirous, leech and Gleditsia fruit that usually dissolved most average-sized cysts in just one cycle. The best way to help yourself when dealing with ovarian cysts is to see an herbalist who can prescribe a special tonic or tincture to meet your specific needs.

Case Study

After suffering with the pain and discomfort of ovarian cysts for years, and ultimately infertility, Carol decided to take drastic measures. She scheduled a procedure to surgical remove a large cyst form her ovary. But, before the procedure a friend suggested that she see an herbalist for a more natural cure. Figuring that she had nothing to lose she did just that and took the herbal treatment described above for three weeks, discontinuing the treatment several weeks before her scheduled surgery. The day of the surgery was a big surprise when a sonogram not only showed no signs of the ovarian cyst, but a growing fetus within her womb!

Endometriosis

Endometriosis is caused when pieces of the inner lining of the uterus begin to grow outside the uterus. Endometriosis usually affects the fallopian tubes, ovaries, bladder, and sometimes even the pelvic cavity found in the abdomen.

About one third of all fertility problems stem from endometriosis, which can cut a woman's chance of getting pregnant by 40%!

Endometriosis may be affecting your ability to get pregnant by:

Blocking your fallopian tubes.
Destroying the fimbraie found in the fallopian tubes that help guide the released egg through the tube.
Causing cysts that may interfere with the egg's release every month.
Creating an immune response in the pelvis that interferes with fertilization.

The good news is that nearly 70% of all women suffering with mild endometriosis do conceive on their own without help – it just takes longer (as much as three years). The rest need some help including surgical IVF or other treatments.

Treatment Options

Although there are several treatment options available to endometriosis patients, there is no cure. Some of the most common treatments include:

Surgery to remove the endo through laparoscopy.
Medications to stop ovulation for a period of time to give the endometrial time to heal
IUI (intrauterine insemination) or IVF.

Of course, you can always try some diet changes, which happen to respond well to endometriosis. One positive dietary change is to try adding plenty of good fats to your diet like flax seed oil and walnut oil, and getting rid of bad fats like saturated fats, butter and lard.

The Eastern Way of Treating Endometriosis

The Chinese categorize endometriosis as Static Blood (or blood stasis with heat or damp heat), that isn't flowing as it should. As the blood remains fixed it creates endometrial cells which the immune system believes should be eradicated. This creates a toxic environment for an implanting egg. Treatment is usually threefold, beginning with a macrobiotic-type diet which is free of dairy, wheat and most animals products to help calm the immune system and its response to the endometrial cells; supplemental therapy to help mute immune responses; and prescribing an herbal formula to clear the internal blood heat and calm the uterus. Acupuncture may also be used.

The herbal treatments for treating endometriosis often have surprising results, with pregnancy occurring naturally within months. Of course, it is imperative that the imbalance causing the body's energy system and organs to go haywire must be addressed. According to TCM, the most common diagnosis patterns for endometriosis include:

Liver Qi Stagnation.
Heat.
Damp Heat.
Blood Stasis.
Cold Conditions
Spleen Qi deficiency.
Kidney Yang Deficiency.
Blood Deficiency.
Mixed heat and cold deficiency.

To be treated correctly, the source of the energy pattern must be detected and treated as well as any hormonal issues.

Fibroids

Fibroids are the most common abnormal growth (tumor) of the female reproductive system occurring in the outer and inner walls of the uterus and the pelvic region. They can be as small as a pea or as large as a cantaloupe. Some women have only one or two, while others may have several, which can interrupt their cycles and cause infertility by either blocking the egg at the uterine cavity or prohibiting implantation.

Western medicine usually treats fibroids with either hormone therapy or surgery.

Eastern medicine, on the other hand, takes another approach: treating the blood stasis which causes the growth in the first place. In most cases herbs are used to invigorate the blood, eliminate stasis and get rid of excess heat, as well as deal with any liver Qi stagnations.

Acupuncture and acupressure can also aid in the elimination of fibroids using the points associated with BI X in the uterus. Stimulating points such as Sp 10 and UB 17 can also invigorate the blood and shrink fibroids.

When you have too much estrogen in your body, benign growths called fibroids can grow inside the wall of the uterus. Fibroids can be a real fertility killer due to the fact that they can change your pelvic anatomy; alter the blood supply to the uterus and even interfere with an egg implanting after it has been fertilized. With more than 25% of all women past the age of 35 suffering with fibroids (many are unaware that they have them), it's no wonder so many couples are finding it difficult to conceive.

When fibroids are suspected, your doctor may order a ultrasound; hysteroscopy, allowing the doctor to insert a small camera through the cervix for a better view of the uterus; HCS or laparoscopy to determine how many fibroids you have as well as how large they are. Depending on their overall size and location, they may need to be removed in rode rot make a pregnancy possible.

Many doctors are now using herbal treatments and acupuncture in conjunction with the surgical methods described above to help treat fibroids. Be careful though when using blood-moving herbs to break down fibroids since they can also cause a miscarriage should conception take place during treatment.

Some other self-help treatments that can be used to help treat fibroids include:

- losing weight (extra fat cells in your body can produce more estrogen)
- eating a low-fat high fiber diet
- eating only organic meat and vegetarian dairy substitutes
- avoiding soy products (it contains an estrogen-mimicking compound)
- eating more cruciferous veggies
- eating artichokes
- detoxifying the body to help strengthen liver function
- improving circulation through exercise
- taking Vitamin B supplements
- limiting sugar and caffeine

- avoiding processed foods

- supplementing with dandelion root, burdock, turmeric and milk thistle

- drink fresh lemon juice to stimulate the liver

- take warm baths with Epsom salts

- adding more omega-3 fatty acids to your diet

- try yoga

- avoid stressful situations (slow down your life!)

When it comes to preventing fibroids in the first place, an emphasis on reducing your exposure to too much estrogen; strengthening the liver to enable it to better excrete excess estrogen from the body and promoting better circulation in the pelvic region are all needed. This can all be accomplished by undergoing a herbal remedy designed to treat your specific issues; losing weight (fat cells increase estrogen in the body; avoiding dairy products which can be very congestive to the reproductive system; Avoid soy which contains estrogen like ingredients; eat a well-balanced diet filled with cruciferous fruits and veggies; stimulate lover function by adding some lemon juice and radishes to your diet; follow a detoxification program designed to clear the liver of excess estrogen; indulge in regular warm baths with Epsom salts and apply castor oil packs to your lower abdomen twice a day during your period (it helps the lymphatic system remove debris from the uterus).

Blocked Fallopian Tubes

Some of the most common causes of blocked fallopian tubes include adhesions, infections, PID (pelvic inflammatory disease), scar tissue, and endometriosis. The number one cause of blocked tubes is a Chlamydia: an infection few women ever know they have.

A tube can be blocked near the uterus or near the ovary. Generally if the blockage is near the uterus, there is a higher success rate with surgery.

Hydrosalpinx, results when a watery fluid collects within the fallopian tube, damaging the far end of the tube, nearest the ovary. It can lessen the effectiveness of various infertility treatments (in vitro fertilization [IVF]). Hydrosalpinx can also be toxic to embryos, with fluid spilling into the uterus. When this is a concern, your doctor may advise you to have the affected tube(s) removed prior to undergoing IVF – the best treatment option for blocked fallopian tubes. Surgery to repair the affected tube may also be considered.

Of course, Traditional Chinese Medicine takes another approach to treating this disorder. TCM considers the fallopian tube the "golden pathway" for the egg to get to the uterus and therefore must be cared for especially well. Since they are so narrow, virtually any infection can obstruct them, leaving the egg little (if any) room to make their way to their destination in the warm, nourishing womb.

Although never easy to open blocked tubes naturally, TCM does offer some options. Herbs are used to invigorate the blood and diminish inflammation. They can be taken orally or even injected straight into the uterus to allow the herbs to flow to (and through) the fallopian tubes directly. However, this procedure, while common in China, is not permitted in the United States.

The most common herbs used to alleviate the network of blood stasis which causes obstructions in the fallopian tubes are myrrh and frankincense since they are some of the only herbs able to reach the deepest meridians, especially when used in enema form.

Stimulating the following acupoints may also help to relieve fallopian tube obstruction: Sp 10, St 30, Zigong, St. 29, Ren 3, Ren 4 and the ear triangular fossa.

When it comes to lifestyle changes, it is imperative that you stop smoking immediately. Cigarette smoking is known to paralyze the cilla, those small hairs found in the fallopian tubes whose job it is to propel the egg forward and through to the uterus.

Fallopian Tube Massage

Fallopian tube massage should only be practiced between menstruation and ovulation. When massaging the lower abdomen, begin at points closely correlated with the tubes, approximately five inches down from the navel and about two inches out from the midline (acupoint St 30). Begin by massaging this area in a circular, clockwise motion (using your fingertips), going outward from the midline of the uterus area toward the ovary, returning to the St 30 site. Apply deeper pressure to areas where you feel a tightness or tension (this may hurt), always massaging outward toward the ovary and back again. End the massage with a pumping motion using the heel of the hand.

Whether a blockage in the fallopian tubes keep the egg from travelling to the uterus; the sperm from getting to the egg or even a fertilized egg from getting to the womb (this is called an ectopic pregnancy), doesn't matter; the fact is infertility ensues. When it comes to fallopian tube issues, there are four main reasons why they may become obstructed, with each needing its own course of specialized treatment:

1. Mucus that is too thick. The mucus in the fallopian tube has an important job – to push the egg forward on its journey to the uterus. Problems can arise, however, when too much mucus is made, actually blocking the egg's passage.

2. Infection and inflammation. The cervix can be a breeding ground for bacteria that can cause the inner walls of the fallopian tubes to swell, making them stick together. This is called pelvic inflammatory disease (PID) and is very common condition among women; although chronic PID can cause lasting fertility issues.

3. Excess Liquid. When the fallopian tubes become inflamed due to bacteria or microbes from the cervix, they can fill with liquid pus, which can block the narrow tubes, making it difficult for the egg to pass through. If this puss builds up enough it can also leak into the uterus where it can create a toxic environment for a growing embryo.

4. Scarring and/or Thickening. Sometimes the fallopian tubes can become thick with scar tissue resulting from chronic infection, previous c-sections

or other surgery and even traumatic pelvic deliveries, which can block the passageway for both egg and sperm.

Blocked fallopian tubes can be treated with a variety of options. Laparoscopy can be very successful in clearing out mucus plugs and other blockages, as can HSG treatments. In cases where the blockages cannot be removed, IVF is a good way to bypass it, allowing the doctor to surgically remove the woman's eggs; fertilize them in a laboratory and reinserting them into the uterus for implantation.

If you are looking for a more natural way to treat a fallopian tube blockage, you can use both herbal medicine and acupuncture to increase circulation to the area and break down stagnate blood and phlegm. Some women also find deep abdominal massage helpful in treating blocked tubes. Other self-help options include:

- using castor oil packs on the stomach (especially if you suffer with scar tissues)
- stop smoking; it impedes the action of the cilia which can keep the egg from moving through the fallopian tubes properly

Cancer and Fertility

The good news is that you have beat cancer and have the chance to become a parent! The bad news is the treatments that helped save your life (surgery, radiation, and chemotherapy) may have also destroyed your ovaries or your spouse's sperm – both necessary components to having a child.

Today, more than ever, medical advances are helping couples who have beaten the odds and survived cancer to beat the odds once again and become parents! But wait, there's more good news: statistics show that babies born to parents who have undergone cancer treatments do NOT have a higher
risk of birth defects or childhood cancer.

A Note to Our Female Readers ...

Of course it is much more complicated for women who have overcome cancer to become pregnant than it is for a man who has overcome cancer to impregnate a healthy partner. Mostly because the woman is responsible for not just getting the egg fertilized, but for nourishing and growing a baby.

Let's take a look at the most common female cancers and the affect it can have on our chances of becoming pregnant in the future.

Breast Cancer

As long as your ovaries are left intact and have not been irradiated, most doctors agree that it is possible to conceive a baby after breast cancer. Most, however, do suggest waiting at least two years after treatment before trying to get pregnant.

Ovarian Cancer

If you've been treated for ovarian cancer with radiation or ovarian ablation, your ovaries will not be able to work properly, which will require the use of donor eggs in order to get pregnant. If you were treated with multiple-agent chemotherapy, there's a good chance you'll go into premature ovarian failure (one third of patients do).

Uterine Cancer

Most times, the only way to treat uterine cancer is to completely remove the uterus. This makes it impossible to carry a child. However, in some instances, the ovaries continue to produce viable eggs that can be implanted into a surrogate.

Cervical Cancer

In some early stage cervical cancers, only part of the cervix is removed, which can make a pregnancy possible, although high-risk.

A Note to Our Male Readers ...

Testicular cancer is the most common cancer found in men between the ages of 20 and 34, with 7,000-plus new cases diagnosed each year. If only one testicle is removed, the other one is more than capable of producing the sperm necessarily for fertilization. However, if both testicles are affected, it's important to freeze several samples of semen prior to surgery to ensure a chance at fatherhood later on.

Some chemotherapy treatments do cause some temporary loss of fertility, usually lasting about three years. Radiation may also deplete sperm counts temporarily.

In the event that ejaculation is affected by the removal of lymph nodes sperm aspiration with ICSI and IVF may be necessary to achieve a pregnancy.

Tubal Ligation

Nearly 40 percent of American women of childbearing age have been surgically sterilized, with at least 10 percent changing their minds later on. Can tubal ligation be reversed? Maybe, maybe not. A lot depends on when the surgery was done and what kind of surgery it was.

If you are considering a tubal ligation reversal, be sure to find a surgeon who specializes in it to increase your chances of success. Not always guaranteed to work, reversal surgery does have some risks:

Scar tissue formation.
Infection.
An increased risk of ectopic pregnancy.

If the fimbriated end of the tube (the part that the egg enters from the ovary) has been left intact and your surgeon is able to reconnect the tube, you may have a higher chance at getting pregnant than a woman undergoing an IVF procedure.

Recurring Miscarriage

In many cases, the same immunological factors and hormonal imbalances that prevent conception are also the cause for a couple's loss of one or more pregnancies. Miscarriage is devastating at any stage, but repeat miscarriages can cause additional strain on the woman's body and the couple's relationship as they struggle to deal with their grief and wonder "why."

One of the most common reasons for early miscarriage is inadequate progesterone production. Using treatments for Kidney Yang or Spleen Qi deficiency can also help to enhance the woman's ability to carry a fetus to full term.

Herbs to improve progesterone production to prevent pregnancy may differ depending on the underlying cause. For instance, if your miscarriages have been due to a spleen deficiency, taking herbs to boost your blood won't help. Here are a few herbal treatments to try for specific diagnosis patterns:

For Spleen Qi deficiency, take Atracylodes (Bai Zhu), Astragals, Codonopis and Dioscera.
For Kidney Yin Deficiency use Encomia bark, Dispacus, Loranthus and Cuscuta.
For Blood Deficiencies try fleece flower root and gelatin.
To clear excess heat from the upper body take Scutellaria.

Some women may find premade herbal formulas for the prevention of miscarriage helpful. They can be found at most Chinese pharmacies and herbal clinics. They may include:

Protect the Fetus and Aid Life Formula – should be used to treat Spleen Qi Deficiency.
Warm the Menses Decoction – used to treat cold uterus.
Cinnamon Twig and Poria Pill – used to treat blood stasis in the womb during pregnancy.
Preventing miscarriage takes a two-fold approach: preparing the body before conception and treating any deficiencies once conception occurs.

Varioceles

Varioceles is a cluster of enlarged veins in the testes that accounts for 40% (or more) of all fertility problems – with these numbers being even higher among men suffering with secondary infertility (meaning that they have naturally fathered at least one child without intervention).

When varioceles occurs, blood that has clotted in the testes can heat the area to over 98.6 degrees, which is at least 1-2 degrees higher than they should be. This can cause serious damage (or even kill) sperm!

Usually only detected through a physical exam (varioceles makes the testes feel like a bag of worms), the disorder is treatable using a form of microsurgery, combined with herbal remedies to increase blood flow through the testes. Be patient though; both treatments take awhile to work. Most patients report a 1-2 year wait until a natural pregnancy occurs on its own.

Testicular Trauma

While we're talking about problems with the testicles, let's discuss trauma. Who hasn't laughed at a comedy show here a man is blasted in the groin? It may look funny on film, but in reality, any blow to the groin can be dangerous. Testicular trauma is considered anything that compromises the blood supply to the area.

This can be anything from a severe blow or certain twisting actions from exercise or horseplay. While keeping swelling down is very important after any injury (use ice packs and anti-inflammatory drugs), more severe cases may require surgery in order to reverse the damage.

Blockage of the Vas Deferens

The tube that moves the sperm from the testicle to the urethra where it is ejaculated into the cervix is called the Vas Deferens. When this small tube is blocked, sperm cannot make their way to where they are needed, which can make conception impossible. There are several things that can cause a blockage of the Vas Deferens:

Surgery: any type of surgery in the groin (hernia repair, prostrate surgery; etc), can all cause Vas Deferens blockages.

Congenital Absence of the Vas Deferens: some men are born without a Vas Deferens tube on one or even both sides of the testes. Depending on the severity of the abnormality, fertility may or may not be reinstated using a surgical repair.

Undescended Testicle: although surgery can be used to descend the testicle, it does not guarantee full fertility function in the future.

Infection: any type of infection can block all or part of the Vas Deferens. The most common culprits of this disorder are: Chlamydia, gonorrhea and tuberculosis.

Orchitis: a viral infection can also cause the testicular to swell, both on the inside and outside. This can also block the narrow Vas Deferens tube. Mumps are one of the most common viral infections that cause this type of infertility in men. In the most severe cases, sperm is not only cut off from this important passageway, but can be killed by the virus.

Appendix 1
Alternative &
Complementary
Medicine

As we've already discussed, there are dozens of ways to enhance your fertility and give yourselves a better chance at conceiving. From acupuncture and herbs to diet and exercise and undergoing invasive medical procedures, there certainly isn't a shortage of ideas to consider. For those interested in learning about some additional "natural" ways to enhance fertility, we've included this brief section to discuss a variety of homeopathic ideas.

Yoga

Traditional yoga offers specific postures, mantras and breathing techniques that can enhance fertility. They work by helping to regulate hormone levels, improve blood and nutrient supply to the eggs, ovaries, fallopian tubes, uterus, testes and even prostate. In addition, they are said to slow the aging process of the woman's eggs.

Patience is key when learning these postures and movements, since they must be taught gradually and progressively. For specific breathing techniques, mantras and positions see a yoga specialist trained in boosting fertility.

Massage

The road to pregnancy can be a stressful one, especially if you are undergoing invasive fertility testing and procedures. Since stress has been proven to inhibit fertility, massage is a great way to alleviate the stress you're under and boost your chances of success.

Homeopathy

Like Traditional Chinese Medicine, general Homeopathy considers the whole person and root cause of conception difficulties in order to treat it naturally. Diet, exercise and specific herbs are used to alleviate concerns and allow the body to work at peak capacity in all areas, including fertility.

Healing the Soul and the Body

If we've learned anything in the previous pages, it's that your body can't always conceive if it is not healthy and strong – physically/ emotionally/spiritually. The fact is, a large number of you who read this book will find comfort and hope in its pages and some new ideas to help you achieve your ultimate goal – but a few of you will not. No one wants to admit that carrying their own child isn't possible, unfortunately a small percentage of couples must.

That certainly doesn't mean that you can't – and won't – become parents. It does mean, however, that you may reach your goal in a new and different way than you had originally thought.

For a few women, adoption is not an option. It's their own offspring or none, and if that's the way you truly feel, than you must find a way to live with your decision.

Regardless of whether you decide to start a family through adoption, or you decide to remain childless, you'll have to deal with a myriad of emotions: disappointment, anger and loss and find a way to feel forgiveness, and hope by learning to let go of old expectations for new ones.

Dealing With Your Grief

Trying to beat infertility can become an obsession for many; taking over your every though, feeling and action. Unfortunately, someday your quest will end: either in the conception and birth of your child; or in despair. Coming to grips with the fact that you can't get pregnant (no matter what you try) is heartbreaking. And it requires taking time out to grieve the loss you've been dealt.

It can be hard for some couples to grieve for something that they've never had. The people around them may not understand the depth of their grief when there has never been a child to be lost. Yet, isn't that the cause of their grief in the first place? The child they yearned for and hoped for is just as real to them as the child another couple held in their arms. Losing the hope of someday seeing their child firsthand can be just as devastating as experiencing a miscarriage or stillbirth. And that's important to understand.

Once you make the decision to get off the fertility treadmill, you need to allow yourselves time to mourn your loss and work through it before you can move forward toward the next stage of your lives – no matter what that stage may be.

Once you've taken the time to step back and work through these intense feelings (and take care of yourself and your relationship), you'll be in a better position to decide your next move. Maybe you'll want to consider adoption or surrogacy or even childlessness. These decisions are completely yours. Just be certain that

Page 317

you understand the ramifications of each and how they'll impact your life and your relationship – now and in the future. Some people can't handle the thought of not being "related" to an adopted child; while others don't care where their baby comes from as long as its there's.

Some women couldn't imagine using another man's sperm to fertilize her egg; or allow another woman to carry her embryo for her. That's fine. You must be comfortable with whatever path you choose to travel.

The important thing to remember right now is that you did nothing wrong and that there are other ways to become a mother if you so choose. Children can enhance a life and relationship like nothing less. Once you become a parent, nothing is ever quite the same. But, deciding to say goodbye to that dream is also an option and one that will not destine you to a lonely and empty life. Plenty of couples experience the joys of family in a variety of other ways despite the void of children in their own home. What's important here is to embrace whatever decision you make and live life to the fullest. There are plenty of experiences out there for you – so grab one and enjoy!

Good luck to you dear reader. No matter what path you travel, may it be filled with love, life and acceptance.

Appendix 2
All About Invitro-Fertilization

Fertility treatments have come a long way over the last several decades since the first "test tube" baby was conceived in England in the 1970's. The process that resulted in that pregnancy and the birth that amazed the whole world was In Vitro Fertilization, which is still the most common assisted reproductive technology (ART) today.

Fertility treatments can be both confusing and costly, with more initials and abbreviations than you could possibly remember and with few insurance companies picking up the tab for these procedures. Understanding In Vitro Fertilization is your first step to making an informed choice about your fertility options.

What is In Vitro Fertilization?

An assisted reproductive technology (ART), In Vitro Fertilization (IVF) is basically the combination of sperm and egg completed manually in the lab and the insertion of this pre-embryo back into the mother's womb. If the mother and father are both able to produce eggs and sperm, respectively, then both will be taken and used to create the embryos that will eventually be transferred to the uterus for implantation. In the case of infertility that impairs the ability of either the mother to produce eggs or the father to produce sperm, a donor may be used to provide these. In some cases, such as genetic anomalies, donors may be preferred by the prospective parents.

While science can replicate nature, it's not quite as simple as getting pregnant the old fashioned way. Because doctors want to greatly increase the chances of a viable pregnancy with each transfer, the mother will take fertility drugs to stimulate her ovaries. This hyper-stimulation will produce many eggs, rather than the one that would normally be released during a regular ovulation cycle. Doctors will carefully monitor the mother's ovulation cycle through ultrasound.

Once the eggs are released, they will be retrieved either through laparoscopic surgery or through a newer technique called transvaginal ocycte retrieval. This process is generally done under light sedation or general anesthesia and most women only report cramping as a side effect of the process.

Fertilization is the next step, and it is completed in the lab under conditions that are as physiologically close to the natural environment as possible. The husband's sperm specimen is mixed with the harvested eggs and insemination takes place. Once embryos have formed, they can be transferred to the mother and the waiting begins. Most doctors will transfer several embryos at once to increase the chances of a viable pregnancy. The chance of a multiple birth is very real with IVF: approximately 25% of IVF pregnancies are twins and 2-3% is triplets. A responsible physician will transfer a reasonable amount of embryos and not put the mother's health at risk with a large transfer.

Once the transfer is complete, blood tests can confirm pregnancy within a couple of weeks, ultrasound at about 40 days from transfer. This is generally the hardest part of the process as the success rates vary from person to person and depend on several factor including health and age.

Who is a good candidate for IVF?

ART is not the first step for a couple seeking fertility treatments. All assisted reproductive technologies are time consuming, expensive and can be physically and emotionally exhausting. While IVF success rates have improved in the last decade, it is still not a sure thing and other avenues should be pursued before choosing IVF. Your obstetrician/gynecologist can and should refer you to a fertility specialist if you have been unable to conceive on your own. You will be given a variety of choices to help you achieve parenthood and IVF might be right for you.

If you have already tried fertility drugs, surgery and artificial insemination; your physician will likely steer you toward IVF as the next logical choice. You are a good candidate for the procedure if:

you have endometriosis
your husband has a low sperm count
you don't ovulate regularly or predictably
the problem lies in the uterus of fallopian tubes
you suffer with unexplained infertility

Age plays an important factor in the success of IVF. As you age, you are less likely to have a viable pregnancy as a result of IVF treatments. If you are between the ages of 35 and 37, the success rate is roughly 25% per treatment. Compare that with the rates for women over 40, which would be 6-10% per treatment, and you can understand why IVF can be such a difficult journey.

Common IVF Protocols

Treating your infertility with IVF will require developing a protocol, or a blueprint/ schedule of how your cycle will be done. It will include the medications you'll be taking and instructions on how to take them; plus the procedures you need to follow throughout the cycle.

Reading your protocol

Many patients receive their protocol only to set it aside – don't! In order for your treatment to work, you'll need to follow these directions EXACTLY as written! All-too-often patients think they'll remember everything the doctor tells them (they don't), or they think their protocol is just like their sister's (it isn't).

However, there are only a few variations of protocols including:

Those for women under the age of 35. If you're under 35 and your baseline hormone levels are normal, your
Doctor could choose to start you on a regulation cycle, which includes starting.
Leuprolide acetate (Lupron) a few days after ovulation. Lupron is used to encourage follicle growth and keeps you from ovulating before retrieval. Instead of stimulating a dominant follicle, like your body would normally do, Lupron allows multiple follicles to develop at the same time.
Some doctors prefer to use a drug called ganirelix, a GnRH antagonist or cetrorelix Cetrotide in conjunction with follicle-stimulating medications such as Lupron. It helps to suppress your LH surge so you won't ovulate before your egg retrieval.
If you're over 35, you may be given a modified Lupron protocol, sometimes called a "stop Lupron" cycle. It entails taking Lupron for just ten days following ovulation and then stopping when you begin taking your stimulating medications. This protocol is used to decrease the suppressing effects of Lupron, which can be detrimental to those over 35 who may be producing fewer eggs.
A natural protocol may also be prescribed, with very little or no medication. This protocol isn't common, but it is used with women who can't handle large doses of medications or may have suffered breast cancer in the past.
In addition, your doctor will likely prescribe gonadotropins, or follicle-stimulating medication, usually taken twice a day, although a daily injection can be used.

What if it doesn't work?

The process of In Vitro Fertilization creates many embryos at once, and these embryos can be frozen for later use. Whether or not your first attempt at IVF is a success, you may be able to use those embryos at a later date. If your first transfer is not successful, most doctors would advise waiting for your menstrual cycle to resume before trying another transfer, generally 2-3 months. If your initial egg harvesting resulted in multiple embryos and your doctor did not implant all of them, you can undergo another transfer process without having to go through the retrieval process again. Similarly, if you are able to sustain a pregnancy after the initial transfer, you can go back to those stored embryos in the future should you want to add to your family.

The Cost of IVF

As we mentioned before, many health insurance policies provide little or no coverage for fertility treatments. Even if your policy does have provisions for infertility, it is essential to understand exactly what is and is not covered under your particular plan. Your doctor's office can only tell you what your co-pays are and are not responsible for understanding the intricacies of your individual plan. Your company's flexible spending account program may be a great way to pay for uncovered expenses related to your fertility treatments because they allow you to use pre-tax dollars to cover medical procedures. Whatever your coverage, be sure to fully understand what is available and what you will be responsible for before you begin your journey. A good amount of preparation will save you from unpleasant surprises and heartache down the road.

The average cost for one cycle of In Vitro Fertilization is just over $12,000, according to the American Society of Reproductive Medicine. Of course, this is a national average and may not reflect the cost in your state or area. The cost can be very prohibitive, especially with insurance covering little to none of the expenses and with a success rate that peaks around 30%. If you are in your late 30's it would not be uncommon to have to undergo several rounds of IVF treatment to achieve a successful pregnancy.

In Vitro Fertilization continues to offer hopeful moms and dads the chance to be parents. The technology and understanding has evolved and improved since that first test tube baby in 1978, and nearly 200,000 babies have been born through the process. If you are choosing IVF, the road may be bumpy ahead, but the destination will be worth it.

SIDEBAR: HCG Instructions

HCG (human chorionic gonadotropins) is a crucial part of your IVF cycle. Given 32 to 36 hours before your egg retrieval; its job is to mature your eggs and prepare them to be fertilized.

By giving patients HCG, your doctor can better schedule your egg retrieval. Otherwise, he'd have to wait for your natural LH surge, which can be impossible to work around.

Timing is everything when it comes to taking your HCG shot. It is essential to follow the directions EXACTLY – even if that means doing it in the middle of the night. If you need to take you injection before 2 am, feel free to mix the solution and leave it on your bedside table. Any later than that and unfortunately you'll need to get up and mix it fresh.

Remember, timing is everything with this injection, so do not delay or miss it; lest you risk waiting another cycle to complete your IVF procedure.

Appendix 3

Chinese Herbs and

Their Latin Names

Ai Ye Folium Artemisiae

Ba Ji Tian Radix Morindae Officinalis

Bai Jiang Cao Herba cum Radice Patriniae

Bai Mao Gen Rhizoma Imperatae Cylindricae

Bai Shao Radix Paeoniae Lactiflorae

Bai Xian Pi Cortex Dictamni Dasycarpi

Bai Zhi Radix Angelicae

Bai Zhu Rhizoma Atractylodis Macrocephalae

Bai Zi Ren Semen Biotae Orientalis

Ban Xia Rhizoma Pinelliae

Bi Xie Rhizoma Dioscorea

Bian Xu Herba Polygone Avicularis

Bing Lang Semen Arecae Catchu

Bo He Herba Menthae

Bu Gu Zhi Fructus Psoraleae

Cang Zhu Rhizoma Atractylodes

Chai Hu Radix Bupleuri

Che Qian Zi Semen Plantaginis

Chen Pi Pericarpium Citri Reticulate

Chi Shao Radix Paeoniae Rubra

Chuan Bei Mu Bulbus Fritillariae Cirrhosae

Chuan Jiao Fructus Zanthoxyli Bungeani

Chuan Lian Zi Fructus Meliae Toosendan

Chuan Niu Xi Radix Cyathulae

Chuan Xiong Radix Ligustici Wallichii

Da Huang (jiu) Rhizoma Rhei (wine fried)

Da Zao Fructus Zizyphi Jujuba

Dan Nan Xing Rhizoma Arisaematis (with pig's bile)

Dan Shen Radix Salviae Miltiorrhizae

Dan Zhu Ye Herba Lophatheri Gracilis

Dang Gui Radix Angelicae Sinensis

Dang Shen Radix Codonopsis Pilulosae

Di Gu Pi Cortex Lycii Chinensis

Di Long Lumbricus

Di Yu Radix Sanguisorbae Officinalis

Dong Chong Xia Cao Cordyceps Chinensis

Du Huo Radix Angelicae Pubescentis

Du Zhong Cortex Eucommiae Ulmoidis

E Jiao Gelatinum Asini

E Zhu Rhizoma Curcumae Zedoariae

Fang Feng Radix Ledebouriellae Sesloidis

Fo Shou Fructus Citri Sarcodactylis

Fu Ling Sclerotium Poriae Cocos

Fu Pen Zi Fructus Rubi Chingii

Fu Shen Sclerotium Poriae Cocos Pararadicis

Fu Xiao Mai Semen Tritici Aestivi Levis

(Zhi) Fu Zi Radix Aconiti Charmichaeli Praeparata

Gan Cao (zhi) Radix Glychyrrhizae Uralensis

Gan Jiang Rhizoma Zingiberis Officinalis

Gan Qi Lacca Sinica Exsiccata

Gou Qi Zi Fructus Lycii Chinensis

Gou Teng Ramulus Uncariae Cum Uncis

Gui Zhi Ramulus Cinnamoni Cassiae

Hai Piao Xiao Os Sepiae seu Sepiellae

Han Lian Cao Herba Ecliptae Prostratae

He Huan Pi Cortex Albizziae Julibrissin

He Shou Wu Radix Polygoni Multiflori

Hong Hua Flos Carthami Tinctorii

Hong Teng Caulis Sargentodoxae

Hou Po Cortex Magnoliae Officinalis

Hua Shi Talcum

Huai Niu Xi Radix Achyranthis Bidentate

Huang Bai Cortex Phellodendri

Huang Jing Rhizoma Polygonati

Huang Lian Rhizoma Coptidis

Huang Qi Radix Astragali

Huang Qin Radix Scutellariae Baicalensis

Huo Ma Ren Semen Cannabis Sativae

Huo Xiang Herba Agastaches seu Pogostei

Ji Nei Jin Endithelium Corneum Gigeraiae Galli

Ji Xue Teng Radix et Caulis Jixueteng

Jiang Huang Rhizoma Curcumae

Jie Geng Radix Platycodi Grandiflori

Jin Ying Zi Fructus Rosae Laevigatae

Jing Jie Herba seu Flos Shizonepetae Tenuifoliae

Ju He Semen Citri Reticulatae

Ju Hua Flos Crysanthemi Morifolii

Ku Shen Radix Sophorae Flavescentis

Lian Qiao Fructus Forsythiae Suspensae

Lian Zi Xin Plumula Nelumbinis Nuciferae

Long Dan Cao Radix Gentianae Scabrae

Long Gu Os Draconis

Long Yan Rou Arillus Euphoriae Longanae

Lu Gen Rhizoma Phragmites Communis

Lu Jiao Pian Cornu Cervi Parvum (extract of boiling)

Lu Lu Tong Fructus Liquidambaris Taiwaniae

Lu Rong Cornu Cervi Parvum

Mai Dong Tuber Ophiopogonis

Mai Ya Fructus Hordei

Mang Xiao Mirabilitum

Meng Chong Tabanus Bivittatus

Mo Yao Myrrha

Mu Dan Pi Cortex Moutan Radicis

(Sheng) Mu Li Concha Ostreae

Mu Tong Caulis Mutong

Mu Xiang Radix Saussureae

Nu Zhen Zi Fructus Ligustri Lucidi

Pao Jiang Rhizoma Zingiberis Officinalis

Pi Pa Ye Folium Eriobotryae

Pu Gong Ying Herba Taraxaci Mongolici

Pu Huang Pollen Typhae

Qi Cao Holotrichia Vermiculus

Qian Cao Gen Radix Rubiae Cordifoliae

Qian Nian Jian Rhizoma Homalomenae Occultae

Qian Shi Semen Euryales Ferox

Qing Pi Pericarpium Citri Reticulatae Viride

Quan Xie Buthus Martensi

Ren Shen Radix Ginseng

Rou Cong Rong Herba Cistanches

Rou Gui Cortex Cinnamomi Cassiae

Ru Xiang Gummi Olibanum

San Leng Rhizoma Sparganii

San Qi Radix Pseudoginseng

Sang Ji Sheng Ramulus Sangjisheng

Sang Piao Xiao Ootheca Mantidis

Sha Ren Fructus seu Semen Amomi

Shan Yao Radix Dioscorea Oppositae

Shan Zha Fructus Crataegi

Shan Zhu Yu Fructus Corni Officinalis

She Chuang Zi Frucuts Cnidii Monnieri

Shen Qu Massa Fermenta

Sheng Di (Huang) Radix Rehmanniae Glutinosae

Sheng Jiang Rhizoma Zingiberis Officinalis Recens

Sheng Ma Rhizoma Cimicifugae

Shi Chang Pu Rhizoma Acori Graminei

Shi Gao Gypsum

Shu Di (Huang) Radix Rehmanniae Glutinosae Conquitae

Shui Zhi Hirudo seu Whitmaiae

Si Gua Luo Vascularis Luffae, Fasciculus

Su Mu Lignum Sappan

Su Ye Folium Perillae Frutescentis

Suan Zao Ren Semen Ziziphi Spinosae

Suo Yang Herba Cynomorii Songarici

Tai Zi Shen Radix Pseudostellariae Heteropyllae

Tao Ren Semen Persicae

Tian Dong Tuber Asparagi

Tou Gu Cao Herba Impatiens Balsamina

Tu (Di) Bie Chong Eupolyphagae seu Opisthoplatiae

Tu Si Zi Semen Cuscatae

Wang Bu Liu Xing Semen Vaccariae

Page 334

Wu Gong Scolopendra Subspinipes

Wu Jia Pi Cortex Acanthopanacis

Wu Ling Zhi Excrementum Trogopterori

Wu Mei Fructus Pruni Mume

Wu Wei Zi Fructus Schizandrae Chinensis

Wu Yao Radix Linderae Strychnifoliae

Wu Zei Gu Os Sepia seu Sepiellae

Wu Zhu Yu Fructus Evodiae Rutaecarpae

Xian Mao Rhizoma Curculiginis Orchioidis

Xiang Fu Rhizoma Cyperi Rotundi

Xiao Hui Xiang Fructus Foeniculi Vulgaris

Xing Ren Semen Pruni Armeniacae

Xu Duan Radix Dipsaci

Xuan Shen Radix Scrophulariae

Xue Jie Sanguis Draconis

Yan Hu Suo Rhizoma Corydalis Yanhusuo

Ye Jiao Teng Caulis Polygoni Multiflori

Yi Mu Cao Herba Leonuri Heterophylli

Yi Yi Ren Semen Coicis Lachryma-jobi

Yi Zhi Ren Fructus Alpiniae Oxyphyllae

Yin Yang Huo Herba Epimedii

Yu Jin Tuber Curcumae

(Zhi) Yuan Zhi Radix Polygalae Tenuifoliae

Zao Jiao Ci Fructus Gleditsiae Sinensis

Ze Lan Herba Lycopi Lucidi

Ze Xie Rhizoma Alismatis

Zhe Bei Mu Bulbus Fritillariae Thunbergii

Zhi Ke Fructus Citri seu Ponciri

Zhi Mu Radix Anemarrhena

Zhi Nan Xing Rhizoma Arisaematis

Zhi Zi Fructus Gardeniae Jasminoidis

Zi Bei Chi Mauritiae Concha

Zi He Che Placenta Hominis

Zi Hua Di Ding Herba Viola cum Radice

Zi Shi Ying Fluoritum

Zhu Ma Gen Radix Boehmeria Nivea

Zhu Ru Caulis Bambusae in Taeniis

www.ingramcontent.com/pod-product-compliance
Lightning Source LLC
Chambersburg PA
CBHW080338290526
45790CB00010B/3744